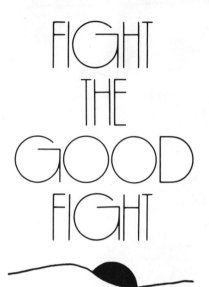

FIGHT THE GOOD FIGHT

FIGHT THE GOOD FIGHT

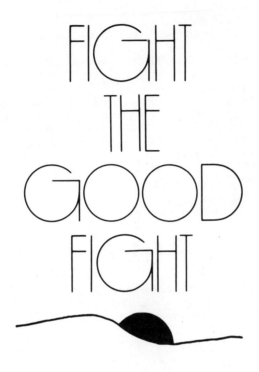

Philip & Joyce Bedsworth

HERALD PRESS
Scottdale, Pennsylvania
Waterloo, Ontario

Library of Congress Cataloging-in-Publication Data
Bedsworth, Philip, 1950-
    Fight the good fight / Philip and Joyce Bedsworth.
       p.   cm.
    ISBN 0-8361-3568-7
    1. Bedsworth, Philip, 1950—Health. 2. Leukemia—Patients—
United States—Biography. 3. Chronic renal failure—Patients—
United States—Biography. 4. Lymphomas—Patients—United
States—Biography. 5. Chronically ill—United States—Biography.
6. Christian life. I. Bedsworth, Joyce, 1950-   . II. Title.
RC643.B42   1991
362.1'9699419'0092—dc20
[B]
                                            91-20148
                                            CIP

The paper used in this publication is recycled and meets the minimum requirements of American National Standard for Information Sciences—Permanence of Paper for Printed Library Materials, ANSI Z39.48-1984.

Scripture quotations are from the *Holy Bible: New International Version.* Copyright © 1973, 1978, 1984 International Bible Society. Used by permission of Zondervan Bible Publishers.

FIGHT THE GOOD FIGHT
Copyright © 1991 by Herald Press, Scottdale, Pa. 15683
    Published simultaneously in Canada by Herald Press,
    Waterloo, Ont. N2L 6H7. All rights reserved.
Library of Congress Catalog Number: 91-20148
International Standard Book Number: 0-8361-3568-7
Printed in the United States of America
Cover and book design by Paula M. Johnson

1 2 3 4 5 6 7 8 9 10 97 96 95 94 93 92 91

To
Sara Joy Bedsworth
and
Steven Philip Bedsworth
You are precious, and we love you.

Contents

Authors' Preface 9

1. White Blood 15
2. In the Beginning 18
3. I Know Who Holds Tomorrow 23
4. Can Dem Dry Bones Live Again? 31
5. Off to See the Wizards 43
6. Bear Ye One Another's Burdens 49
7. God Be With You Till We Meet Again 55
8. Life in the Cocoon 63
9. Coming Home 78
10. Starting Over 83
11. Two Steps Forward, One Step Backward 89
12. The Dark Night of the Soul 93
13. Dying to Live 107
14. Each One's Life Is But a Breath 117
15. When You Pass Through the Waters 123

The Authors 127

Authors' Preface

This is the story of one family's struggle with chronic illness. Over a period of three and a half years, doctors discovered that Phil had leukemia, kidney failure, and lymphoma. Our family has faced bone marrow transplant, dialysis, kidney transplant, and chemotherapy.

There is a significant difference between *acute* illness and *chronic* illness. In acute illness, the disease is resolved. The patient either recovers or dies. In chronic illness, the affliction may be controlled or in remission; it is never gone. Acute illness demands courage. Chronic illness requires perseverance.

Phil does not remember many of the events that follow. He was too sick. The text printed in italics comes from the journal Joyce kept from 1986 to 1989. Through her journal, Joyce managed and interpreted the stress of those days.

What prompted us to write this book? One motive was selfish. Writing provided us with the opportunity to make sense of chaos.

As Phil's illness progressed, one medical emergency followed another. Unexpected surgeries. Life-threatening infections. Fractured vertebrae. Congestive heart failure. Hypertension. We channeled all our energies into facing the crisis at hand. Time blurred. Fatigue settled in. There were few occasions to step back and reflect.

We are now able both to retell these events and to interpret their impact upon family, our friends, and our understanding of how God works in this world.

Writing these words has been traumatic and therapeutic. Traumatic in that we were reminded of our jagged feelings of anxiety, anger, weariness, and grief. Therapeutic in that we could celebrate the many miracles we received and the many caring people who contributed to our recovery.

We wrote this book because it was a story we needed to tell. And we wrote it because we had a message which needs to be heard.

One part of the message looks outward. Modern technology, even as it expands the boundaries of life, places on us the burden of decision. At what point do we stop attempting to prolong life by postponing death? Which medical ethics apply when large amounts of limited resources are poured into one person? How can patients and physicians become partners in health care rather than antagonists battling for control? How does one prepare to die?

Our encounters with medical personnel and institutions are representative. Some were good. Some were bad. We offer them to inform you and to allow you to anticipate your responses in similar situations.

The second part of our message looks inward. This book is our witness to the sustaining power of God and the unfailing love of God's people. One by one illness removed the conventional resources people rely on—self-sufficiency, financial security, structure, and routine.

It seemed we were losing everything, yet we were never alone. God was always present, although often hidden by the storm. God's people stood with us, even when we were surrounded by the darkest of shadows.

Our experiences are not the witness we might have chosen. They are the witness we declare and the faith we invite you to embrace. We are not experts. We do not have all the answers. We are experienced. We hope our story can be a resource to you in your time of testing.

Special thanks to the readers who lovingly critiqued our story in its early stages: Roger Gingrich, George and Arlene Mark, Harold and Mary Weaver. Alvin and Gertrude Blough freed up time for writing by supplying delicious suppers once a week during the spring of 1990.

While Phil was hospitalized in Iowa City, our children, Sara and Steven, needed a surrogate family. Carl, Mary, and Kelly Wiebe moved into our house and into their lives. During this same period, Royce and Eileen Roth opened their home to Joyce so she could be available to Phil in the hospital.

Phil would not be alive today without the life-giving gifts of Beth Bedsworth, Kenny Wilson, and hundreds of anonymous blood donors. Our parents, James and Grace Eicher, and Curtis and Evelyn Bedsworth, were unfailing in their encouragement and their concern. The Hesston Mennonite Church and many other churches across the country supported us with their prayers and their finances.

Finally, we remember our support group, without whom we could not have fought the good fight: John and Jan Blosser, Gerry and Ruth Epp, Ron and Patrice Flaming, Gordon and Delores Funk, Phil and Vicki Hoffman, David and Darlene Myers.

—*Philip and Joyce Bedsworth*
Hesston, Kansas

White Blood

I was preparing for bed on October 1, 1986, when I found it. A lump in my abdomen. Gas? No, the lump was only on my left side.

I turned to my wife, Joyce, and asked, "What is this?"

Joyce, a master's-trained registered nurse, laughed and explained, "These are your ribs. Here is your hip bone. This? I think you're going to have a baby!"

I rolled over and fell asleep. Joyce knew this was not a laughing matter.

The next morning my "baby" was still with me. A full day of pastoral tasks awaited me at Hesston (Kansas) Mennonite Church. Joyce, however, insisted that I see a doctor. We scheduled an appointment for 2:00 p.m. at Axtell Clinic in nearby Newton, Kansas.

After taking a brief medical history, doctors sent me to the lab for blood work. The doctors became less talkative and we more apprehensive.

The silence was broken by the blood report. My

white blood count (WBC) was two hundred fifty thousand. Normal levels are five thousand to ten thousand. My platelet count should have been between three hundred thousand and five hundred thousand. The lab report was over one million. All symptoms pointed to leukemia.

Leukemia. White blood. A disease afflicting sixty-five thousand Americans each year, many of them children. No known cause, no easy cures.

The doctors left the room to arrange an appointment with an oncologist, a cancer specialist. Joyce came over to my chair and sat on my lap.

My first tearful words were, "Don't bury me in Kansas." The Hesston community had been gracious to us, but it was not yet home.

Home was still Elkhart, Indiana. We had lived there ten of our fourteen years of married life. Elkhart was only two hours west of the farm where Joyce's parents lived in Pettisville, Ohio. Elkhart was only two hours north of my parents' retirement home in Berne, Indiana. Now eight hundred miles separated us from parents and siblings. A flight out of Wichita or fifteen hours on the road would normally tame that distance. These would not be normal times.

We would meet the specialist in Wichita on Friday, October 3. Doctors cautioned us that a splenectomy, removal of the spleen, might be necessary. In parting they counseled, "Go home, pack, and wait."

It was late afternoon. The Kansas skies were darkening, both physically and emotionally. We were not ready to face the children. What would we say to Sara, age eight, and Steven, six? We stopped at the home of longtime friends Ron and Patrice Flaming. There was not much to say, only lots of hugs and tears.

We arrived home and decided not to tell Sara and Steven about my illness until we had some firm information. Sara, however, overheard one of our telephone conversations. She realized something was terribly wrong with Daddy and ran screaming into the living room.

We told the children I had a blood illness and might have to go to the hospital. Sara, immediately recognizing that I might die, broke into tears. Steven, only six, was puzzled. How could I be sick when I was standing right in front of him?

By evening other friends found their way to our living room. They assured us we would not walk through this valley alone.

Wearily we headed for bed. Twenty-four hours earlier I had been in the prime of life. I was happily married with two wonderful children. I had completed my education and was moving toward the peak of my career. We were not rich, but we had enough disposable income to buy things on our wish list.

Suddenly all this had changed. Life was not indefinite and open-ended. Death appeared imminent.

In the Beginning

I was born in Philadelphia, Pennsylvania. Dad was pastor of an inner-city church. Mom was an elementary school teacher. In my early years she stayed at home with my younger sister, Beth, and me.

In 1967, Dad retired from the ministry. We moved to Berne, Indiana, my mother's hometown. The next year I entered Goshen College, a school sponsored by the Mennonite Church in northern Indiana. I did well in the classroom but not in campus social life. Insecure, I compensated by being an obnoxious loudmouth.

At the beginning of my sophomore year, I met a transfer student, Joyce Ann Eicher. Joyce had grown up in Pettisville, Ohio. Her father, James Eicher, was a dairy farmer. Her mother, Grace, had her hands full raising six children and running the household.

Joyce, as second oldest, became "daddy's boy." She cut hay, fed pigs, drove tractor. Perhaps being midwife to farrowing pigs ignited her interest in nursing.

Joyce first enrolled in a two-year nursing program at

Hesston College (Kansas). She showed promise in the classroom and was encouraged to consider a four-year nursing degree. At the beginning of her sophomore year, Joyce transferred to Goshen College.

Our first impressions of each other were mixed. Joyce had gained thirty pounds at Hesston; I thought she was fat! Joyce was put off by my severe acne. Second impressions were different. During that fall Joyce and I both did volunteer youth work. I liked Joyce's spontaneity and contentment. She knew who she was and where she was going.

Joyce impressed me. I impressed her—but in the opposite direction. Over the next few years, Joyce broke up with me six times. My loud behavior embarrassed her. She could enjoy me as friend but nothing more.

The turning point came when Joyce decided no one would love her as much as I did. On August 20, 1972, we had an outside wedding on Joyce's family farm, between the house and chicken coop. Like many couples then, we chose a nontraditional service. Our special music was a congregational hymnsing. We had no attendants and composed our own vows.

This is what we promised each other on a hot August afternoon:

> Joyce, I take you for my wife, now, and for as long as God grants us life.
>
> I want to be your best friend and lover.
>
> I promise, with your help, to found a Christian home where love for God is taught and practiced.
>
> I will try to be a leader in our home worthy of your respect and faithfulness.

I will honor you, appreciate your selflessness, and love you as I love myself.

• • •

Phil, I need you to complete my life.

Today I take you to be my husband. I give myself to you to be your best friend, your lover, and the mother of our children.

Each day we have life, I want to share your heartaches, your joys, and your disappointments.

I promise to try to fill each day of your life with joy as we seek God's will for our lives together.

We graduated from Goshen College in 1972. Joyce earned a B.S. degree in nursing; my degree was in English education. That fall I attended the Associated Mennonite Biblical Seminaries in Elkhart, Indiana, while Joyce gained clinical experience on a medical floor at Elkhart General Hospital.

From 1973 to 1975, we lived in Puerto Rico, doing Voluntary Service for the Mennonite Board of Missions. We were unit leaders for a household of thirteen young adults. Joyce began as a part-time nurse at the fifty-bed Hospital Menonita. By the end of our service term, she was director of nursing. I taught junior high English and Bible at Academia Menonita Betania, a small, parochial school for students in kindergarten through ninth grade.

Our service experience fostered in me a fresh interest in biblical studies. We returned to Elkhart, Indiana, where I completed my master of divinity degree at the Associated Mennonite Biblical Seminaries in 1977.

Then we moved to Kalona, Iowa, where Joyce enrolled in the graduate nursing program of the University of Iowa. While she worked toward a master's degree in medical-surgical nursing, I taught high school Bible and Spanish at Iowa Mennonite School.

Nineteen seventy eight was a watershed year for us. Joyce's thesis work required a move back to Elkhart, Indiana. I became pastor of Prairie Street Mennonite Church, with about 250 members. On May 24, Sara Joy joined us. We had been an infertile couple, so Sara's arrival ended five years of frustrated dreams. Sara gained a brother on July 26, 1980, when Steven Philip was born.

We soon discovered that Steven was a chronic, severe asthmatic. His breathing steadily deteriorated, requiring four or more hours of treatment daily. On three different occasions, mucus plugs clogged his airways, precipitating life and death crises. We learned to live with the possibility that we might lose Steven.

Opportunity unexpectedly beckoned from the West. Hesston College invited me to help begin a two-year pastoral ministries program. This allowed me to test whether teaching was what I really wanted to do. Joyce was also invited to join Hesston's nursing faculty.

We taught at Hesston College for two years. I enjoyed the classroom but missed long-term congregational relationships—sharing in births, weddings, crises, and funerals. Joyce also enjoyed students, but discovered she preferred health care administration.

In July 1986, I became lead pastor of the Hesston Mennonite Church, with a membership of six hundred. Joyce began working on her second master's degree in health administration at Wichita State University. Sara and Steven were third and first graders at Hesston Elementary. This was the calm before the storm.

I Know
Who Holds
Tomorrow

On October 3 we had our first appointment with Dr. G. Our first impressions were that he was too young, too encouraging, and too controlling.

Dr. G. performed a bone marrow biopsy on me. He inserted a large needle into my hip near the belt line, extracting a small amount of bone marrow. This test would confirm the diagnosis and indicate what kind of leukemia we were dealing with. It would also reveal how far my illness had progressed.

Six people squeezed into the examining room to assist with the biopsy. Fearful tears would have been appropriate; instead, I found myself laughing. My behind had not received so much attention since I passed potty training. This was only the first of many show-and-tells.

The biopsy confirmed that I had chronic myelogenous leukemia (CML). The presence of the "Philadelphia chromosome" made diagnosis certain. Between 20 and 30 percent of leukemia patients have this type of leukemia. In some forms of leukemia, the white blood count drops to dangerous levels. In CML the bone marrow produces excessive but ineffective white blood cells. The threat posed by all types of leukemia is the inability to fight infections.

CML has three stages. Stage one lasts from three to five years following diagnosis. Stage two, the accelerated stage, lasts about six months. Stage three is the blast crisis. Ineffective white blood cells, called *blasts*, take over the blood stream. The body is left defenseless.

My initial diagnosis was stage one, with the three to five year prognosis. Having feared a quick death, this seemed a long time. We had time to invest in the children. Time to put our financial house in order. Time to complete at least a few of our dreams.

News of my illness spread through the Hesston community. Lack of accurate information set off a rash of rumors. I was in surgery. I was in intensive care. I was dead. A new worry surfaced: would others fear I was contagious? Could I continue working? Should I continue working?

In many cases, people in crisis withdraw. The pain of failure, the embarrassment of illness is not for public display. This would not be our choice. We wanted to be open and honest about our situation. We needed the church to be a fellowship of prayer and caring.

We decided to make a public announcement in church on Sunday, October 5. During the seventy-two hours following diagnosis, the words to an old hymn *I Know Who Holds Tomorrow* came to mind. We wanted to use them in our announcement but could not recall all of the words. Who had a copy of the lyrics?

The hunt in the church music library was futile. Our need triggered a community-wide scavenger hunt. People searched in home libraries, checked attics, and scanned old hymnbooks.

Finally our neighbors Robin and Mavis Lowrey located an old phonograph recording of the song. We transcribed the words that would guide us through the next three years:

> Many things about tomorrow, I don't seem to understand.
> But I know who holds tomorrow, and I know who holds my hand.

On Sunday morning tension filled the sanctuary as we approached the pulpit. No one knew what to expect. Impulsively, I yanked open my suit coat and proclaimed, "See, I'm all here!"

We reported what we knew about my condition. We asked the congregation to walk with us and to pray for us. That Sunday happened to be Worldwide Communion Sunday. My legs buckled as Joyce and I walked forward to receive the bread and the cup.

The next day, October 6, was my thirty-sixth birthday. I woke up wondering if I would ever see a fortieth birthday. Cards came in surprising numbers. Friends made us a pizza-size birthday cookie. Our Sunday school class decorated our front lawn with luminaries placed to form a giant thirty-six.

My best birthday present was a note from Milo Kauffman, president emeritus of Hesston College. Milo had quickly perceived, not only the burden of our situation, but its potential blessing as well.

No doubt you had been looking forward to a long life of service to Christ and to his people. Christ said, "No, Phil, you and Joyce are my chosen vessels for short-term, special service.

"It may be as witnesses of my healing power. It may be as witnesses to my all-sufficient grace in affliction and suffering. The trying of your faith will be more precious than would be an ordinary life of service."

May your testimony be like that of the apostle Paul:

"Unto us is this grace given: that we should be God's chosen vessels to witness to his love and grace to his people."

Milo did not say God was punishing me. He did not say God chose us because we could handle it. He simply affirmed that God's hand was with us. Our situation, seemingly so oppressive, could be an opportunity to let our little light shine.

Milo's words of comfort fostered a dream—to show my sisters and brothers, to show the world, how a Christian faces death. That was the dream. I also had a nightmare: that in my time of testing, my light would flicker.

Shortly after my diagnosis Joyce began keeping a journal. The journal was her quiet place, her refuge from the chaos and confusion that engulfed us. Here she would name her fears and pen her hopes for my life and our life together.

10/12/86 THESE DAYS when I read literature about this leukemia and when I'm away from Phil, I feel overwhelmed, anxious, and scared. When I think of all the love, prayer, and concern shown by God's people, I just know everything will be okay. Details are fitting into a better order. But making phone calls for Steven's night-time medication and child care still seems hard. We are learning more and more about the preciousness of life.

10/12/86 THIS WEEK *Sara has wanted to be surrounded by her friends. She wants to forget what's going on. Teachers at school feel both children are in denial.*

Wednesday evening after Joy Bunch supper, Sara wanted Rachel to come home with us, even though it was after 8:00 p.m. She just does not want us to be alone together as a four-some. It's too painful. On Saturday she was extremely irritable—picking fights, not cooperating, demanding to play games with Daddy and the whole family.

She denies any fear about Daddy's illness. She did admit that she wakes up thinking about Daddy. Sara likes to be with her friends because this helps her forget her sad feelings. I told her I was available to talk with her whenever she want-ed.

Sara's teacher will be calling later tonight to report her ob-servations. On Thursday I wrote a note to Sara's teacher to find out how Sara was doing.

Sara said, "Mom, this is the third time this week that you sent a note to school. Soon people are going to think that we have family problems."

I said, "Do you think we have family problems?"

She quickly replied, "No," and went out the door to school.

Now Sara and Steven are in the bathtub together laughing. Phil is completing my paper on the word processor. I'm feel-ing very scared, as if life may change drastically, afraid that Phil will die soon. I give him a hug as a tear slides down my cheek. Even if a bone marrow transplant works out, the stress, pain, and anguish will be great in the coming months.

If it doesn't work out, how can I live without him?

10/14/86 LORD, IT *seems there is so much to do and so little time in which to do it. I feel I'm really living to the full. I feel deep pain as well as the warmth of your love and care. I find great joy in small things—a kiss, a hug, a tooth coming out, and many things to laugh at. Thanks for your presence, Lord.*

10/20/86 WHAT WILL *the outcome of our story be? Only you know that, Lord, only you. These past weeks you have held us closely in your arms. You have surrounded us so beautifully with your people. You have heard so many thoughts on our behalf for Phil's health.*

You know Phil is your servant. You know he loves to preach about you and your love. You know that in life or death he is yours; yes, he is yours.

It's comforting to know that when he leaves this earth he will be with you. We joke about him calling me thirty minutes each day from heaven. Then I think I can make life here on earth.

What will it be like for me to be single again? You know how I nearly cry when these thoughts run through my head. This weekend we celebrated Phil's birthday with Hoffmans and Swartleys at a restaurant. Last evening our Sunday school class played baseball together. Will I still be welcome when I'm only half a couple? Who will I be without Phil at my side? We've learned and loved to be quite the team, you know.

10/20/86 THANKS, LORD, *that Phil is not physically hurting and is psychologically strong. We continue to share many tears, wondering about our tomorrows. Yet I firmly believe that it is only today I can live. I need to enjoy it fully. Phil, Sara, Steven, people, work, play, leaves—all of your creation.*

Help me to find the balance in all of this so that I don't get too tired.

Thanks, Lord, for the special time we had yesterday playing Monopoly with Sara and Steven. They are trying to be so brave. Sara has become sassy. She's talked with Phil about the fact that Steven seems to get more of his time than she does. Help us, Lord, to show her how special she is to us and how to give her special time.

The benefit of cancer, if there is one, is the opportunity to say goodbye. Heart attacks and car accidents bring life to an abrupt end. There is no time for farewells, no time to tie up loose ends.

How would we spend my last days? Well-meaning friends encouraged us to take a last fling: a cruise, a cross-country trip, something exotic. Others suggested quitting work and concentrating on family.

I indulged my love for gadgets by upgrading my computer with a color monitor. But doing strange and extraordinary things was not appealing. We wanted to treasure the ordinary and routine. This meant staying home and continuing to work.

Diagnosis had been made. The bad news had been shared with family, friends, and church fellowship. Now came the tedious part. We entered the rhythm and rigors of chronic health care. Acute health crises are intense, but short-term. The patient either recovers or dies. Chronic illness lingers.

Our lives were no longer our own. Our schedule revolved around doctor's appointments and lab work. Our trip from Hesston to Wichita took about ninety minutes round trip. We invested hours traveling back and forth on interstate I-135. On arrival, we sat long hours in waiting rooms, both anticipating and dreading the doctor's directions.

I quickly grew to hate my weekly blood tests. It was not only the bee sting of needle insertion. It was the unavoidable reminder that I was sick. These tests, however, were the best indicators of what was happening to me.

The initial results of chemotherapy were encouraging. There was a steady decline in my white blood count, from a high of two hundred fifty thousand to a near-normal thirteen thousand. This decrease was good, but we knew that the chemotherapy was only treating symptoms, not causes. Treatment could slow the progress of the illness, but it could not cure me of leukemia.

Can Dem Dry Bones Live Again?

The only hope for long-term cure of my leukemia was a bone marrow transplant. Bone marrow produces blood. Once marrow begins producing bad blood cells, the process cannot be reversed. The original marrow must be completely destroyed. New marrow must be introduced and engrafted into the patient's bones to begin producing healthy blood cells. Cure for leukemia and related blood diseases is truly a life-and-death experience.

Several risks accompany the transplant process. First, the patient is vulnerable to the slightest infection. As the old marrow is destroyed, there is nothing with which to fight disease. Consequently, it is a secondary infection, not the leukemia, that usually causes death.

Second, the patient (host) may reject the new marrow (graft) leading to graft-versus-host disease (GVHD). This can be minor, resulting in a skin rash easily treated with a therapeutic cream. GVHD can also produce major gastrointestinal upset or lethal damage to essential organs. GVHD seems to be age-related. The older the patient, the less adaptable he or she is to new tissue.

Finally, there is the trauma of treatment. There is not yet a standard protocol for bone marrow transplant. Each medical center develops its own treatment program. Even with these diverse approaches nearly every patient suffers the breakdown of not only one but multiple body systems. The transplant process is so demanding that in 1986 few centers would do bone marrow transplants on patients over forty. At thirty-six I was already pushing the age limits.

The key to successful transplant is the match between donor and recipient. The closer the match, the less chance of rejection or GVHD. The ideal donor would be an identical twin. The next best donor is a sister or a brother. Some medical centers are experimenting with unrelated donors. Their success rate at this point is low in comparison to related donors.

Even a sibling is not an automatic match. Each sibling has a one in four chance of matching with another sibling. I had but one sibling, my sister Beth. She was thirty-four, single, and teaching junior high English in Elkhart, Indiana. If we did not match, we could consider one of my parents as donors, but that would have been a move of desperation.

When we approached Beth with our need, she was both eager to help and apprehensive. She had had little experience with hospitals other than a tonsillectomy at age eight. The match process would require extensive blood tests and on-site interviews at transplant centers. As donor she would undergo surgery and general anesthesia. Recovery from surgery was not expected to be difficult, but no one could guarantee what her individual response would be.

Beth consented to be my bone marrow donor, assuming that we were a match. This was no small gift to offer, even for a brother.

We began the extensive—and expensive—match process. Testing comes in two parts. The first test, human leukocyte antigen (HLA), checks whether there is a compatible match. The second test, mixed lymphocyte culture (MLC) further defines the level of compatibility.

Joyce had predicted that Beth would be a compatible donor. She was right. Both the HLA and the MLC were matches. We had successfully crossed the first hurdle in bone marrow transplant.

10/23/86 IT HAPPENED! The phone rang and it was Dr. G's office. Phil and his sister, Beth, are a "full house match." This is the best match possible. Excitement and fear gripped my body. Now a bone marrow transplant is an option—but, oh, the risks.

Most people have no comprehension of what this means. Phil has a chance for cure. He could also die soon.

The door to bone marrow transplant was open—but should we walk through? Coincidentally, Joyce was in the middle of a medical ethics course at Wichita State University. Each class session reminded her of the limited health resources available and the number of patients denied care when such resources are poured into a handful of complex cases. What right did we have to consume enormous amounts of health care resources for a highly risky attempt to forestall death?

In addition, we anticipated a worst case scenario: that I would survive bone marrow transplant, but in a severely disabled state. We wondered, "Would it be better to savor life and then die quickly and, hopefully, quietly?"

10/31/86 LIFE STILL seems to be going too fast. Last evening I began a course in "Issues in Health Care." In today's class people who make federal and state laws spoke to us. One person, who administers Medicare services, said that funding six liver transplants would mean cutting services to twenty thousand persons currently receiving funds. She named the programs that would go—those to keep elderly in their homes, to keep children healthy, and to provide prenatal care for teenage pregnancies. Impressive! Who should get health care?

These economic realities prompted additional ethical questions. As Christians could we justify heroic efforts such as bone marrow transplant to avoid death? What did our faith mean in this time of medical crisis?

The questions related to bone marrow transplant evaded easy answers. We turned to the church for help. I had always preached mutual accountability in decision making. Now we had a chance to practice it.

We put together a fact sheet for the Hesston congregation which we distributed on October 28. We identified the tremendous financial costs of bone marrow transplant. We explored the prospects and burdens of long-term disability.

Bone Marrow Transplant (October 28, 1986)

We face a very difficult decision. At the time of Phil's diagnosis, doctors told us that he might be a candidate for a bone marrow transplant. Such transplants are only done on persons younger than 40. That hope seemed remote. A "match" needed to come from a full brother or sister. Each sibling would have only a one in four chance of matching. Phil has only one sibling—a sister, Beth, who is a remedial reading teacher in Elkhart, Indiana.

The *good news* is that we have discovered that Phil and his sister, Beth, are a match. The *difficult news* is that a bone marrow transplant is a very risky procedure. There is a 45 to 50 percent chance of a "cure" from leukemia. There is a 25 percent chance that leukemia will remain active. There is a 25 to 30 percent chance of death occurring during the transplant process.

Such a decision brings many emotions to the surface: fear, excitement, and hope. It also poses medical and ethical dilemmas.

Last weekend was a well-timed retreat for Phil and me. We had time to think about what this option might mean for us. This morning we invite you to be part of our decision-making process:

1. In the past weeks, we have discovered that Phil's disease has progressed further than we had first thought. It is amazing to me that he seems so well. However, no one knows just how and when he will become ill. It may be a few weeks or several months.
2. We know that Phil's kind of leukemia will enter a final stage, called *blast crisis*. When this happens, there is little that can medically help. Once the acute stage begins, death usually occurs within two months.
3. A bone marrow transplant is the only medical offer of

cure. Phil would need to be in good physical condition, with his leukemia as controlled as possible. He must still be in a chronic state, rather than the final stage. This means we cannot wait long if we choose this direction.

Our doctor is saying we should plan to do the bone marrow transplant shortly after the holidays. This seems very soon.

At first, I thought I could not bear to look at living without Phil so quickly. Perhaps some of you are feeling that now. Because you have remembered us with your thoughts and prayers in so many ways, I am now open to looking at a bone marrow transplant. God, through God's people, gives great strength to face very difficult times.

4. We have *not* yet made any decisions about a transplant. We will be going to Mayo Clinic sometime in November to gather more information.

   We do know some things now. If we go ahead with a transplant, Phil and I will need to move to a transplant center for about three months. Sara and Steven would remain here in Hesston. Such a family separation is extremely difficult for us to consider.

   We would need your help: to take care of the children, to assist with Steven's asthma care, to support the caregivers with meals and weekend breaks. Additionally, we would need people to watch over the house and our financial matters. Most importantly we would need prayers, prayers, and more prayers.

   To keep you informed, a call tree would need to be set up so that you could have accurate, up-to-date information.

5. The process of bone marrow transplant will involve heavy chemotherapy and radiation therapy. This means Phil will be *very* sick. He will lose all his hair

and be very susceptible to *all kinds* of infection. He will be placed in a sterile room with special air ventilation.

The actual receiving of the transplant is rather simple. It is much like getting a blood transfusion. The problems come before and after the transplant.

6. Even a "successful" transplant carries major dangers. The long-term risks include the following:

   a. Infection—a major threat to life for at least six to twelve months.

   b. Bleeding, leading to hemorrhage.

   c. Graft-verses-host disease—in which the transplant tries to reject the recipient's body. This can affect many body systems for years after the transplant. It can also result in death.

   d. Possibility of leukemia returning.

We know of two other people who had the same kind of leukemia Phil has. Both had transplants. Both died within two weeks of the transplant. One of them, Tony Wyse, was a friend I grew up with. His story is available from Jane Friesen (church secretary) in the church office. In addition, copies of what we are saying this morning are available on the platform.

We outline the pros and cons of this decision so you can pray with and for us. This is a life-and-death decision. Should we enjoy the days and months left to us? Or should we try this risky procedure and perhaps hasten Phil's death in hope of a cure?

If we decide on a bone marrow transplant, we must be prepared both for the end of Phil's earthly life and for a fresh gift of life.

We believe that God, through the prayers and medical skills of his people, can grant physical healing. *We* do not know God's overall plan, but *God* does. We are sure it is a good one. We know that spiritual healing *will* take place.

We have asked four couples to help us in the decisions

we face. They are Gordon and Delores Funk, Phil and Vicki Hoffman, David and Darlene Myers, and Ron and Patrice Flaming. In addition, our Sunday school class has been and continues to be a place where we can share thoughts and feelings. As you pray, talk, and think about this decision, share your thoughts with one of these people or with us, perhaps as a written note.

We have been deeply touched by the overwhelming response we have received this last month in response to Phil's illness: phone calls, letters, cards, visits. Many of you have shared with me tough moments in your own lives. Many of you have lost loved ones, either through death or divorce. You have survived.

There *is* hope. *You* have made it through. That means I can, Sara and Steven can, Hesston Mennonite Church can, the broader Mennonite church can.

God has been very good to us. God's family is a great one and one which we are proud to be a part of. I thank each of you for being who you are. You are very special to us.

Our plea received mixed reactions. For some, there was no issue to debate. If there was hope, seize it! Others were appreciative of our candor, but did not know what to say. Giving counsel on the church budget was one thing. Giving counsel involving a life-or-death decision was something different.

No one wanted to offer the wrong counsel. The most frequent response was, "We will support you, whatever direction you take."

10/28/86 OH GOD, I'm scared, scared, scared. My heart is full of fear and this feeling has not gone away for several days. The decision regarding bone marrow transplant looks incredibly big. The loss of Phil seems too much to bear. The way to long-term recovery carries with it the risk of losing him very, very soon.

We must finish planning for Phil's death before we can look to the future and the hope of a bone marrow transplant. Much as we try to live these days normally, they are not and will not be normal for some time. We need the routines in our lives right now. Too much quiet time feels far too heavy.

To make a complete decision, we realized our need for more information. In Beth we had found the right donor; now could we find the right bone marrow transplant center? Someday bone marrow transplant will be a science; for now it is an art. Procedures differ and success rates vary. Experience is a key factor in patient survival.

Where to go? We began to educate ourselves about options. We read popular pieces on bone marrow transplant. Joyce secured research articles on mortality rates and complications. We learned that Seattle was the American pioneer in bone marrow transplants. They had the most experience; they also had a lower survival rate than other centers.

We narrowed our choices to three centers. Dr. G was promoting Mayo Clinic. He argued they were the best and he himself would go there. It was also true that he was a Mayo alumnus. Under his prodding we agreed to a November 25 visit.

Our second option was not one we sought; it was given to us. On Saturday, November 1, we received an unexpected call from Royce Roth, then chairman of the Hesston College Board of Overseers. News of my illness had reached him in Iowa City. Did we know that the University of Iowa Hospitals and Clinics had a bone marrow transplant program? Did we know that Roger Gingrich, a Mennonite physician, managed it? Would we call Roger that night?

That phone call was crucial. Roger was competent, compassionate, and concerned that we act quickly. Our shared Mennonite faith and heritage made conversation flow easily. We arranged for an on-site visit on November 19.

Our third option also came about through church connections. We became acquainted with Berdon and Jenise Epp from Henderson, Nebraska. Berdon had received a bone marrow transplant at the University of Nebraska Hospital in Omaha. He was pleased with the care he had received. Our phone conversations with physicians in Nebraska were positive. But we chose not to visit Omaha.

11/02/86 YESTERDAY EVENING we talked with Roger Gingrich, who is a Mennonite transplant physician working at the University of Iowa. He confirmed some of what we were told but also shared his experience and practices. He indicated that at best Phil's life expectancy is short!

11/03/86 LITTLE STEVEN has broken my heart much of this evening. He talks about his fear of Daddy dying. This makes his throat sore and his tummy sick because he feels so sad inside.

I told him that we too have thought a lot about Daddy's death and have cried a lot. That is okay.

I also told him that Daddy might get better! His former baby sitter, Amanda Fast, had a brother, Berdon Epp, who re-

ceived a bone marrow transplant and he is doing well. He is a daddy again to his two children.

Steven just sat in the car looking sad and hugging Sara's stuffed animals Freckles and Patty. He said that in music class today they sang "It's Okay to Cry." They sang it even though Steven is in first grade and "it's a second grade song."

Steven told his class about his daddy's illness. They all said his daddy didn't look sick. I told him that when we visited the transplant centers that I would take some pictures of the kind of room Daddy would be in.

Tonight at bedtime Steven was again saying how sad he felt. Then he asked if he could pray. "Help my daddy to get well again. Help Mommy with her homework. Help Sara to catch up in math and help me to catch up in math. In Jesus' name. Amen."

We talked about the possibility of his talking and praying with the school counselor tomorrow. He thought that would be a good idea.

As I was leaving his room, Steven said, "I think Daddy should have the bone marrow transplant even though it is risky. He might do okay or he might die, but I think he should do it."

Bless his little heart. He thinks too much and knows too much. He just needs lots of hugs right now.

Sara just tries not to think about it. It will be interesting to see how she works through all of this. I hope she can unload her burden on someone. She is so very sensitive.

11/10/86 TODAY I WENT to the cemetery with Ron Litwiller and Phil. Being there today at time of sunset didn't seem so bad. Maybe that will be where Phil's body will rest. He wants a tomb stone like Opal's, a former member of Hesston Mennonite Church, with an engraved gladiolus like the one I carried in our wedding. We would carve, in addition, the life verse we chose on our wedding day: "Trust in the Lord with all your heart and lean not unto your own understanding. In all your ways acknowledge him, and he shall direct your path."

11/11/86 OH, GOD, is this all going to work? Will we get to be a family of four? You have been near us in so many ways. Just now, calm the storm inside of me. We love you and want to serve you as best we know how.

Off to See
the Wizards

We woke up on November 19 to a Kansas ice storm. We had arranged to fly in a college plane to Iowa City with Hesston College flight instructor Glen King. We discovered at 6:30 a.m. that the plane was not equipped for ice flying. Our hospital appointment in Iowa City was scheduled for 9:00 a.m. How could we possibly meet our deadline?

I paced up and down the airport hanger as Glen tried to make alternate flight arrangements. At some subconscious level, I knew that my days of health were numbered. To reschedule our appointment in Iowa City would mean losing precious weeks in initiating treatment.

Glen made contact with Don Horst, a member of our Sunday school class and owner of a charter flying service. Don graciously made special arrangements to take us to Iowa City. To our great relief we were only fifteen minutes late for our appointment.

The University of Iowa Hospitals and Clinics is the

largest medical center in Iowa and the largest teaching hospital in the United States. Royce Roth met us at the airport and escorted us to Clinic B.

Despite the size of the university hospitals, we did not feel lost. Roger Gingrich was a gracious host, and the nursing staff on 7 Carver East treated us with respect and concern.

Roger suggested we repeat the bone marrow biopsy done in October. The results were not good. We had believed I was in the initial stage of CML. This new biopsy indicated I was well into the second, accelerated stage.

I did not have three to five *years* to live. I had three to five *months*. If we were to take action, we needed to do so immediately.

11/24/86 ONCE BACK in the aircraft, fear gripped us. Were we too late for a bone marrow transplant?

We've worked hard these past seven weeks to prepare for Phil's possible death or life. Suddenly the game seems to have changed. Our time for life together is even shorter than we anticipated.

I felt so sad as we held each other and cried.

11/24/86 THIS MORNING Steven crawled in bed and snuggled his little butt up next to me. I love those kids so much. What will separation be like for all of us?

Today at our front door was a special gift—a koala bear to give us all hugs from Gerry, Ruth, Lisa, Sonja Epp. What gift to show their love. The kids both wanted to take it to school to share at share time, so there was a fight.

Steven settled the issue just moments before Lowerys picked them up for school. Sara would have it first and Steven would go to her room later to get it.

Steven asked whether we had decided if Daddy would have the bone marrow transplant.

I said, "We want to, if doctors say it can still be done."

Steven continued, "Good, 'cause then someday Daddy can give me rides on his legs again. Until then Carl [Wiebe] can do that."

I wish Sara could talk more. I'm going to take her out alone sometime and hold her, hug her, see if she will talk. She reacts by fighting, crying, and demanding I do things she can do for herself. These are the hardest behaviors for me to deal with.

I wish we could talk about her hurts. I'm sure some of my responses hurt her, yet I know she has such tender and caring thoughts and feelings.

The selection of a transplant center took on new urgency. Our initial contact with Iowa City had been so positive that we questioned the need for the trip to Mayo Clinic. However, we decided the comparison of medical centers would confirm or redirect our choice.

The sky over the Rochester, Minnesota, airport was gray, the air chilling. My first impression was that this frozen wasteland was not the sort of place in which I wanted to die. The clinic had requested that my sister Beth join us to complete blood studies. My mother accompanied Beth, both for moral support and to see me.

Our experience at the clinic was frustrating. We moved from one enormous waiting room to another. We were disappointed that the primary issue in our interview process seemed to be money: who would pay for this bone marrow transplant? This was a legitimate financial concern. Initial costs for a bone marrow transplant in 1986 were $125,000.

Our interview with Dr. Z was scheduled for 1:00 p.m. We were still in the waiting room at 2:30 p.m., wondering about our 4:00 p.m. plane departure. This time pressure colored our interview. We never seemed to connect with Dr. Z and regretted we had not chosen Omaha for our second scouting visit.

11/25/86 I FOUND Dr. Z difficult to deal with. He seemed to question us at several places, as though he did not believe us. He seemed indifferent to our questions. Instead, he lectured us about CML and bone marrow transplant.

If only Dr. Z had taken time to listen to us! Instead, he kept telling us we needed to make a decision about bone marrow transplant. We had already decided to attempt a bone marrow transplant. Our question was where!

We had made our scouting trips. Now it was time to decide. We evaluated medical statistics, support services, and the resources offered by local churches. We chose Iowa City. In a few weeks, we would become adopted Hawkeyes.

We had a match. We had a center. The season for decision making had ended. Now it was time to fight the good fight in earnest. An uncertain future loomed before us. We could approach it as helpless victims; we chose to be survivors. Our lot was to deal with an unfair and hostile environment. We would do battle with all the creativity and imagination we could muster. Some battles we would lose. We would try to win the war.

The battle demanded that we be clear-eyed and single-minded. It would consume our physical and emotional reserves. It was an all-out fight for life. Wishful thinking about a magical cure or a new wonder drug was a thinly disguised form of denial. There was no quick fix. There was no frontier tonic "good for what ails you."

Before we could fight for life we had to face death directly. We reviewed our legal responsibilities. Car titles and property deeds were properly written "with right of survivorship." We discussed trust funds and investment counselors. Joyce took over household accounts so there would be no surprises after my death.

We updated our wills. Kansas law requires the executor to be a state resident, forcing an adjustment in our will. Anticipating some difficult medical situations, we drew up a durable power of attorney. The power of attorney clarified who had authority to make decisions about heroic interventions on my behalf.

We examined our choices regarding guardians for the children. The first time we had written our wills, this step was a technical necessity. Now guardianship was a central concern.

To whom would we entrust our children? Our original choices had been close friends. We looked at family dynamics, speculated about parenting styles, and re-examined shared values and priorities.

We decided to ask Joyce's sister Jeannette and her husband, Vernon, to be guardians for Sara and Steven. We knew Sara and Steven would never be lonely with them—not with five cousins to contend with!

Like many young families, we had given little attention to funeral planning; now we had reason to do so. Joyce was overwhelmed by the thought of planning my funeral in the instant of loss. My pastoral experience confirmed the pain of decision making under traumatic conditions.

Through the generosity of Roger and Lou Ann Eichelburger, church friends, we spent a weekend at a Holiday Inn in Wichita. Freed from our parental responsibilities, we wrote funerals for the four of us.

A funeral deserves the careful attention we give to a wedding. It is a time of remembrance, celebration, and farewell. A funeral is also an opportunity to make a final statement of faith.

We resisted the temptation for an exaggerated eulogy while conceding the need of others to speak. It was important to me that there be congregational singing. My suggestions for a sermon text focused less on tomorrow and more on today: the abiding presence of God even when storms rage and rivers run wild.

We anticipated the milestones at which death would deny my presence—graduations and the wedding days of our children. We pushed back the shadows by writing letters for those occasions. I can think of nothing more painful and gut wrenching than composing those letters. I sobbed deeply as I envisioned those special moments and my empty chair.

Bear Ye
One Another's
Burdens

Hesston Mennonite Church continued to lovingly support us, as did congregations across the country. Now, however, we needed something more. We needed persons to help us with the nitty-gritty action steps.

We drew together a small support group. Four couples agreed to walk through the valley with us. They were Ron and Patrice Flaming, Gordon and Delores Funk, Phil and Vicki Hoffman, and David and Darlene Myers.

These couples struggled with us as we sifted through our medical choices. Their insights helped us avoid hasty or incomplete decisions. They were our liaison to the church and the broader community.

The support group also faced with us the practical problems of long-term, two-to-three-month hospitalization. Chief among these was child care. Joyce and I had decided that we would leave the children in Hesston. We would not have the emotional energy to parent them as we would want. Further, keeping their friends and school routines seemed a prudent course when everything else was so uncertain.

Sara was eight years old, Steven six. Who could be their surrogate parents? Who could provide the love and patience they would need during this uncertain season? Steven was a chronic, severe asthmatic, requiring several hours of specialized therapy each day. Who would accept such responsibility?

Many people wanted to help us, yet no one felt able to take primary responsibility for Steven. My associate pastor, Carl Wiebe and his wife, Mary, stepped forward. Mary was an R.N. willing to walk the medical tightrope with Steven. Carl and Mary, with their one-year-old daughter Kelly, offered to move into our house and be mom and dad. It was a gift few others could offer.

With the help of our support group, we organized the community to help Carl and Mary with their responsibilities. There was a massive mobilization of volunteer resources. Various families signed up to bring in meals. Some agreed to help with house cleaning. Others volunteered to be on call to help with Steven's treatments, especially in times of acute need.

Our cries for help were graciously answered by the people of Hesston. Sara and Steven would receive the best care possible. Still there was a price to be paid. We would never know the laughter, the anger, the fears of those months. They would grow dramatically and we would only watch that growth from afar.

12/01/86 FRIDAY IS another day of mazes. The kids were home from school. I found myself short tempered. I felt like a failure as a mom. I knew they needed extra care, but being told they needed a drink and being expected to get it ready for them seemed too much.

After eating at Pizza Hut, Sara and I made party mix and snickers bars. As I was mixing something up, I looked over and she was crying. I held her on the couch, and we talked about how life might change.

If Phil died, Sara did not want a new daddy. She wanted to know what would happen to the three of us. Would we move? What would life be like if Daddy did live? All these were difficult questions to look at.

We held each other close and talked until the phone rang. It seemed she was then ready to cook again. We were very tired and soon off to bed.

Other issues besides child care required attention. We would be ten hours away from home. Who would pay the bills? Who would maintain the house? Who would answer the questions of a worried community?

The support group agreed to shoulder these responsibilities. They would take over our checkbook—talk about accountability! They would screen our mail. They would be the contact people for medical updates and concerns. They would take over every important aspect of our lives.

We could leave Hesston on fifteen minutes notice knowing all local needs were covered. We could be single-minded in our fight for life.

Even while we planned for life I was preparing to die. I stopped buying clothes. What sense was there wasting money on items that might soon go to the local thrift shop? I agonized over who should get my professional library. I lost interest in the news and we canceled the morning paper.

I noticed an increase in daydreaming. How should the epitaph on my gravestone be worded? I fantasized farewell conversations with friends near and far. I played and replayed my deathbed scene, which usually resulted in tears and sobbing.

We began to think in detail about the hospital stay. The average hospitalization for bone marrow transplant patients is six to eight weeks. Several of those weeks would require isolation. People would be able to enter my room but I could not leave it.

The bone marrow transplant unit on 7 Carver East had a number of double rooms for patients. This would help, but still those five walls would grow steadily smaller. How could we make an institutional room home? Roger and the bone marrow transplant staff encouraged us to move in—and we did.

Home for me meant my computer. As long as I could think, I would try to record the events of these days and their meaning. Home also meant books. We naively packed three boxes of Bible commentaries and theology books. I did not complete reading a single one.

No place could be home without music. My little stereo system would fit snugly next to my bed, accompanied by a favorite tape of hymns sung by the Kansas Mennonite Men's Chorus.

By the time all this was loaded, it made quite a pile—almost too much for our little Ford Tempo. Even as we packed, the shadows crept close: would Joyce need to lug all this stuff home by herself?

My toys and books were important. But home, more than anything else, meant the faces of the people I love. We had a treasure trove of informal photographs which Joyce assembled into a montage. Like many young families, however, we had few formal portraits or family sittings. To postpone pictures could mean an empty place.

We contacted Don Gering, a member of our Sunday school class and a professional photographer. He provided us with a wonderful selection of close-ups and family shots.

As an invitation and a reminder for prayer support, we had Don make up five hundred copies of our family picture. We distributed these to the congregation and other interested persons across the country. Eventually the picture appeared on the cover of the June 1987 *Christian Living,* a family magazine published by the Mennonite Church.

I am not a formal person. Joyce wanted one picture that reflected that informality. We moved into the study where it took me ten minutes just to clean off my desk. Don posed me, feet on desk, computer at hand, reading the weekly magazine of the Mennonite Church, *Gospel Herald.* The resulting portrait was not dignified, but it was honest.

One step of preparation remained. My housing and personal needs would all be supplied by the hospital. What would Joyce do? It was not just a matter of a place to sleep. Joyce needed access to cooking and laundry facilities. She needed a place to rest and to recover from the stress of the day. Joyce needed people with whom to laugh and to cry.

Iowa City is home to the University of Iowa. As in any college town, housing is tight and expensive. The cost of renting a motel room for two months was prohibitive. Finding an apartment would be tricky and living there would be lonely.

Royce and Eileen Roth solved our dilemma. They lived a mile from the hospital. Their three children were all grown and married.

Joyce was welcome to a bedroom and bathroom for as long as I was hospitalized. Royce and Eileen would provide housing, mealtime fellowship, and a listening ear when things got tough. The Roths' home remains our home away from home.

God Be With You Till We Meet Again

Arrangements for child care, finances, and housing were now complete. It was time to prepare my body for bone marrow transplant. Roger explained that my spleen, still greatly enlarged, was a reservoir of leukemic cells. My chances for successful transplant would improve if doctors removed it. The surgery was scheduled for St. Francis Regional Medical Center in Wichita on December 2.

The course was set. It was time to let go of my pastoral responsibilities. On November 30, the first Sunday of Advent, I gave my farewell sermon. I did not know if it was also my final sermon.

My closing words were ones of reflection and hope.

God has been walking with us. God has been walking with *all* of us. He has not told us why. God is teaching us to wait in hope.

We are being taught discernment. You and we have made fresh decisions about what is important. We have made fresh commitments to our marriages, to our families, to our God.

We are being taught compassion. Throughout the past two months, we have never felt isolated. We asked you to walk with us and you have. It is the business of God's people to take care of one another. We are being fashioned into a community of care.

We are being taught how to pray. We ask, "For what am I praying?" We ask, "To whom am I praying?"

It is encouraging to see God's people gather in prayer. It is humbling to be the one prayed for. It is exciting to watch God bring healing.

We don't yet know if God will bring cure. God *is* bringing healing and wholeness, just as God did twenty centuries ago.

Dr. B performed my splenectomy on December 2. He also inserted a double-lumen catheter in my chest. Through the catheter, staff could extract blood samples and administer blood transfusions. Over the next two months, this catheter would become a dear friend.

Recovery from the splenectomy was uneventful—but not for long. Surgery was Tuesday morning. By Wednesday afternoon, I was feeling terrible. When nursing staff took me to the bathroom, I passed out. Someone had missed some vital signs. I had lost four units of blood. I was in shock and in serious trouble.

12/04/86 It seemed like forever since I had last seen Phil. I was surprised by the way he looked. He seemed so pale. They had just hooked up his IV to his Raaf catheter. He had a warm feeling in his chest, followed by a pressure.

Phil was nauseated. At 1:15 p.m. I walked to the nurse's

station to ask for something for nausea. This did not seem all that unusual since his nasogastric tube, a tube leading into the stomach, had been removed this morning. Phil continued to feel warm. To me he felt cool and moist, especially from the elbows up. His pulse was 140 and thready, although the student nurse got it at 80. Phil was restless.

I lowered his bed and finally, at 2:00 p.m., he got a shot for pain. The nausea continued. Still no shot for nausea was given. No one took a blood pressure.

The Raaf catheter was irrigated and found to be open with correct position. At 2:25 p.m. Phil vomited old blood. I pressed the call light but no one came. I asked the student working with the other patients to get help and an emesis basin. She walked slowly so I asked her to hurry.

Seven minutes later our student nurse came in. She seemed surprised that he had vomited. I asked her to get another basin, which she did. I asked her to measure and save the emesis because it was old blood. She did not seem concerned about it.

Finally I said, "I want it saved and checked by a staff nurse because it's blood."

She said, "Well, I don't know what it is. I've never seen it this color."

I replied, "Then I'm telling you—it's old blood!"

In the course of this fiasco, I discovered that no one on the floor had ever worked with a Raaf catheter before. This did not boost my confidence in Phil's nursing care.

I should have stayed with Phil. I feel so bad that I didn't. Never will I sit back like this again.

I returned to the operating room for my second surgery in twenty-four hours. My abdomen was full of blood, but no bleeder could be found. Doctors concluded that my platelets, while numerous, were ineffective. The good news was that the bleeding had stopped. The bad news was that we could go through the same trauma all over again, with no warning.

I was transferred to the eighth floor, medical intensive care unit. Staff referred to this unit as the "arm pit of the hospital" because of its age and run-down condition. What a delightful place to recover!

12/07/86 I DON'T understand this kind of incompetent care. I questioned my own observations because I was told all was normal and no one paid much attention to the situation. I did not want to cause major problems.

What should be done about this event? Yes, we have talked to physicians, nursing administration, and friends. Is this enough? Do we forget what happened? I can't do that just yet.

Hardest for me to accept is that this crisis is a result of incompetent nursing care. Major errors were made by a student nurse, a student instructor, and a staff nurse—my peers and colleagues! It makes me cry just to think about it.

Yes, the bleed would have happened anyway. What could and should have been different is early treatment of the bleed. With good nursing care, the physicians could have been informed earlier. They could then have ordered medical care to correct the situation. Phil might not have gotten so sick.

A great learning for me: even if a person is hospital staff, I will not trust decisions which conflict with my thoughts.

Dr. B decided to leave my nasogastric (NG) tube inserted until things settled down. Imagine a small hose stuck through your nose and down your throat. The NG tube was necessary but a great nuisance.

I was emotionally devastated. I became obsessed with the fear that another bleed would ambush me. I determined to stay awake—all the time.

By Thursday night I was sliding into "ICU psychosis." I saw myself falling into giant marshmallows arranged like teeth. I knew that if I landed, I would die.

I begged for Joyce to be in the room, even though it was 2:00 a.m. I cajoled the nurse into walking me at 4:00 a.m. As if some demon were at work, my overhead fluorescent light began burning out.

When it seemed nothing else could go wrong, Dr. G came into my room. He casually—but catastrophically—mentioned that Beth and I were an MLC (mixed lymphocyte culture) mismatch. In short, she could not be my donor for bone marrow transplant.

When we pressed him for details he replied, "We'll talk about this later."

All our planning and hopes had been based on a match with Beth. Had all our work, including the splenectomy, been in vain?

The near fatal bleed, the news of MLC mismatch, and extreme fatigue combined to overwhelm Joyce. She went home to recover for a few hours. I was left alone in my room. My only companions were my nurse's button and that stupid nasogastric tube. It was a terrible morning, worsened by a flickering fluorescent bulb and the lack of a clock.

Joyce returned that evening renewed. So was I. David Myers and Gordon Funk had sat with me that afternoon. The nasogastric tube was finally out. Gordon had also brought me a clock with which to mark time.

On my release from St. Francis Regional Medical

Center, we contacted Roger in Iowa City. What were we to do? Roger believed the reported MLC mismatch was an error. He urged us to repeat the tests using the Iowa City labs. This time my parents would also be tested to get as complete a genetic picture as possible.

We eagerly agreed, recognizing the additional expense and trauma this meant for Beth, my parents and us. Roger soon called us with good news: Beth and I were an MLC match, although it was the narrowest of matches. We were a one-way match. Beth could be a bone marrow donor for me, but not I for her.

Once more we anticipated a bone marrow transplant. The double surgery had been a major setback for me. The transplant, originally set for mid-December, was pushed to January. I had to rebuild my stamina or the transplant would be difficult.

Joyce and I started walking—and walking. The Yost Center, the athletic center on Hesston College campus, was a great resource in winter weather. By the end of December, we were walking six miles a day. I was even able to play a few games of racquetball!

12/13/86 I GOT UP *at 6:30 a.m., showered, and then started Steven's treatment. Sara usually gets up around the same time (although today she slept until 7:22 a.m. Boy, was she angry with me.).*

She was sassy the whole morning, angry at everything I said or did. She said she wanted to get her own breakfast.

I said "Fine!" and then she didn't want to. She hated her shoes and it was my fault, even though she had picked them out. I had to turn and laugh.

This is not my usual Sara. It's good she can get some anger out. Both Phil and I were tempted to call the school to see if they noted behavioral changes. For so long she seemed not to show this stress. Wow! Now it's anger, pure and simple.

Lord, help me show her I love her and understand her anger.

12/14/86 OUR CLASS papers were due today at Wichita State University. Other students asked about my plans for next semester. I keep saying I don't know what's ahead.

I find it difficult to think ahead to tomorrow and make plans. The only relevant concern in my life is today. I don't know what tomorrow will bring. I only know that today we are a family of four in Kansas.

There are so many things I want to do—but how do I organize them? Do I clean, water plants, prepare Christmas cards, clean off my desk, decide what to take to Iowa? I forget.

Today I take time to sit by Phil and talk and open mail with him. I wonder, "What if he is severely disabled?" I just hope for the strength to live each day.

12/17/86 STEVEN AND I talked. He said he felt as if he had no friends. He felt really sad about the trouble he and Ben got into at the ball game on Friday evening. A principal yelled at him because they were playing under the bleachers. He just sobbed and sobbed. I felt so bad for him. He wants to be with Mom and Dad and never go to a friend's house again.

Steven says he doesn't like school. I asked if he would like to talk with Duane, the school counselor. He thought that would be good.

What will the emotional cost of this crisis be? Who will be the casualties? Can I survive this pain? What if Steven really doesn't have friends? What positive steps can I take?

12/18/86 TODAY STEVEN had an appointment with his pulmonologist, Dr. Lucht.

On the way Steven said, "Mom, if in the future—I'm talking about the future—if Daddy dies, kids at school won't be able to treat me and Sara bad. I'll feel too sad to finish my work or even play."

Steven said he was already different because he had asthma. No one else does a treatment. He is the littlest one in his class—"because of steroids." His daddy is sick and might die. No one else has that. I felt sad inside. He has a pretty good understanding of how things are.

This morning I had a conference with the school counselor and with Steven's teacher, Mrs. Loganbill. This conference took almost one hour but it was time well spent.

Steven spends much of his time lying down or seated at a table by himself. He often does not participate in recesses. No wonder he doesn't feel he has friends. He simply does not interact with others.

Steven will be moved to a large table with other kids. He will be expected to do the same activities. Sometimes the best thing to do is what seems cruel. At the same time he needs many hugs and support to assure him he is a fine kid.

Christmas 1986 was not easy. We followed our traditional patterns. We set up the Christmas tree on Thanksgiving Day. We mailed Christmas cards. We bought Christmas gifts and wondered what secrets their bright-colored wrappings held. Below the surface happiness one question haunted us all: was this our last Christmas together?

We splurged on the kids. Their presents were more extravagant than any other Christmas in their young lives. I did not want them to lack anything. I wanted them to remember this Christmas—and me.

Life
in the
Cocoon

It was time to go. On January 3, 1987, we packed the car for Iowa City. Joyce and I took a final stroll around the house. Here were the shrubs and bushes we had planted. Here were the walls I had spent a summer scraping, priming, and painting. Here was the little metal playhouse we had built for Sara and Steven. Would I see this house again in this life?

Sara and Steven had stayed overnight with David and Darlene Myers. Their children, Rosanna and Ben, were the same age as ours. We hoped that having play-mates would ease the pain of separation.

We found Sara and Steven playing in the upstairs bedrooms. Our arrival seemed an interruption to their games. We hugged all around, said good-bye, then walked out the door.

Tears streamed down my cheeks as we drove to-ward the interstate exchange. Had my good-bye been a final farewell? There were so many things to teach them, dreams to nurture, milestones left unshared.

*01/03/87 W*ITH *A few exceptions Phil and I have faced this challenge together, encouraging and caring for each other. He's made me happy. I feel I've made him happy too.*

Now we are off to a new adventure, a life of radical changes. What lies ahead? Newness of life? Disability? Death?

Lord, we love you. We will keep believing that you will care for us no matter what the outcome.

We traveled north on I-35 through Missouri, then east on I-80. By nightfall we were in Iowa City. Royce and Eileen were gone for the weekend but had insisted that we stay in their home anyway. What a gift! We did nothing dramatic. We avoided last minute adventures. We were content to be quiet and alone.

My stamina and strength were eroding but I did not feel sick. I realized this could all change in seventy-two hours. My journal of January 4 reflected my mood.

> Different people have asked me about my life review. I feel fortunate to have enjoyed a good marriage for over fourteen years. I have had more marital joy and sense of partnership than many people with forty years of married life behind them.
>
> I have achieved a measure of success in my career—both as a pastor and as an instructor at Hesston College.
>
> I have had the chance to parent two wonderful children.
>
> If my life ends abruptly in the next few weeks, I will be disappointed, but I cannot say I will feel cheated.

On Monday morning, January 5, we checked into the University of Iowa Hospitals and Clinics. I became patient 86-33252-8. On the bone marrow transplant unit (7 Carver East) there were rooms for about ten adult patients, divided into two "pods."

Directly across from my room was Bob, who had received a bone marrow transplant about four months earlier. Following his transplant, Bob suffered a stroke. He was confused and incontinent. I watched his wife walk him down the hall, clothed in his diaper. Bob incarnated all my worst fears about bone marrow transplant.

Just down the hall was Jake. He held the record for the fastest release from the transplant unit—twenty-two days. He had returned to the hospital with a suspicious respiratory infection.

Joe was in the room next to mine. He had returned to the hospital following transplant with an acute infection.

The bone marrow transplant unit practiced primary nursing. One nurse would coordinate my nursing care and be my liaison with the medical staff. Deb introduced herself as my nurse and made it clear I would not be babied. I would do my own personal care, clean my chest catheter, and in general take care of myself. In hindsight, this strategy of enabling patients to take care of themselves is an effective means of maintaining morale and encouraging recovery.

I went through typical admission procedures: medical history, lab work, chest X-ray, pulmonary function (breathing tests), and a fresh bone marrow biopsy. As a reward for my day's labors, I received a sixteen-hour home pass. Shopping at K-Mart never felt so good!

Initial lab results Tuesday morning indicated a blast

count of 19 percent. This meant about one-fifth of my white blood cells were ineffective. Had we missed our window of opportunity for bone marrow transplant? With great relief, we received a revised count on Tuesday evening of 9 percent blasts.

The numbers meant we had used up my good days. We were at the right place, with the right people, at the right time.

01/06/87 DOCTORS LINQUIST and Miller made rounds. They informed us that the preliminary blast count in bone marrow was 19 percent, higher than we had anticipated. Phil is clearly in the accelerated phase. The report surprised us because peripheral blood counts had seemed so good.

After the doctors left, we went for a walk feeling sad and disappointed. We were so hopeful that Phil's illness was still in the chronic state. As we walked, the thought came to me, "At least we aren't throwing away good days. We are at the brink of life's end for Phil.

"Whether or not we proceed with the bone marrow transplant, he will get very sick soon. With the transplant there is some possibility of life; without it there is none."

Lord, be merciful to me. Help me find my way through life's maze. I trust that many people are also praying for our families and close friends. The grief of this loss will be felt in a wide arena, but so will the joy of Phil's healing.

I received my first dose of chemotherapy on Tuesday evening, zero day minus nine. Beth's marrow would be transplanted on day zero. Each day until transplant, I underwent either chemotherapy or radiation treatments. The goal was to destroy every single colony of leukemic cells in my body. If even one colony remained, chances were high for a recurrence of leukemia.

Saturday, zero minus five, was *cytoxcyclophosphamide* day, a particularly toxic chemotherapy. To avoid damage to healthy tissue, medical staff insert a bladder catheter to help flush out the medicine.

On Monday, zero minus three, I began my radiation therapy. Chest or dental X-rays last less than a *second*. I would undergo six *hours* of total body radiation, equivalent to all my sunshine for the rest of my life.

I was alone in the radiation room, monitored by closed-circuit television. Each treatment lasted an hour. I lay on my side and tried to hold still.

I played cassette tapes as the radiation attacked my bone marrow. I chose *Godspell* and *Jesus Christ Superstar*. The interplay of crucifixion-death-resurrection themes and my own struggle was emotionally staggering. Tears flowed freely as I pictured the cross and the sacrifice Jesus had made on our behalf. Would my Golgotha lead to an Easter morning?

Finally it was January 15, day zero. Beth had been admitted to the hospital the night before. That morning she went to surgery, where six large needles were inserted into her hip area. Through these needles doctors harvested two units of bone marrow.

At the time of my transplant, the transplant team was using several different protocols for bone marrow transplants. In my case, they took Beth's marrow and removed as many T cells as possible. The theory being tested was that a decrease in T cells would decrease the chances of rejection or GVHD (graft-versus-host disease).

Jim Radford and Jeff Miller, fellow and resident respectively, entered my room midafternoon with the treated marrow. This was "the transplant."

The procedure was no more complicated than a blood transfusion. Jim and Jeff connected an IV tube to my chest catheter. A special filter in the line screened out small blood clots. In about two hours the process was complete. No trumpets, no blinding lights, just the transfer of one life to another. The transplant opened the door for a new life. Could I walk through?

That night we had a "zero" birthday party with family and our Iowa support group. We feasted on homemade birthday cake and three flavors of Schwann ice cream. It dawned on me that from now on I would have two birthdays to celebrate each year—my birth on October 6, and my rebirth on January 15.

We lit a blue candle as a symbol of new life and hope. Over the next year, we would light an additional blue candle each week to mark my progress toward health. When we reached fifty candles, the heat of one candle would melt another!

Parties and candles were only part of our hospital survival tactics. The bone marrow transplant unit had a VCR. We took full advantage of it. Like Norman Cousins in his book *Anatomy of an Illness*, we used laughter as an adjunct therapy.

One of our favorite movies was the Mel Brooks' comedy *Blazing Saddles*. In one scene, a group of cowhands is eating beans around the campfire. The normal consequences of bean-eating ensued. The next day I passed gas for the first time since my bone marrow transplant. We cued the movie to the campfire scene and offered this to my doctors as my daily progress report.

All bone marrow transplant patients await their blood counts, evidence that the new marrow is engrafting. We turned the counts into a sweepstakes. We gave poster prizes for those who could guess the date when my white count or platelets reached self-sustaining levels. For the grand prize winner, a sitz bath with the patient of her choice! Corny? Yes. Childish? Perhaps—but effective.

Were we blind to the gravity of our situation? No. Fellow patients were always slipping into serious and often fatal infections. However, we rejected the myth that life is hopeless. To be sure, we had our moments of panic and despair, but we refused to surrender to the Shadow-Keeper.

Until the new marrow began producing blood cells, I was totally dependent on blood transfusions, as many as three a day. Each night around midnight blood samples were drawn from my catheter. I frequently woke up to find a unit of packed red blood cells or platelets hanging on my IV pole.

These blood products were gifts of life from strangers, persons I would never know but people who cared. They were gifts from people who, whatever their background, answered God's call to stewardship and compassion. Beth had given me an essential gift, but without these other, anonymous gifts, her contribution would have been in vain.

01/21/87 GOD, SURROUND and protect Phil's body. The dark circles around his eyes remind me of how sick he is.

God, make it as easy as possible for him. Protect him.

Help us maintain a positive attitude surrounded by and uplifted by your love through other people. No matter what the end, I'm grateful for this time together.

01/25/87 HOW STRANGE *our living arrangements are. I'm lonesome to go home, be a mom, and have our family intact and together.*

Mary and Carl sent a letter and called about several problems with Steven. One is night-time wakefulness. Our doctors have said in the past that breathing problems can awaken kids even though they don't seem to be in major difficulty.

In my imagination I see Steven going off to his room himself, sobbing quietly, then starting to cough and vomit. Perhaps we have babied Steven too long, but so often his fears, breathing problems, whatever, go away if we are near.

Lord, be very near to Steven and surround him with your love. I can't be there just now, and I want to be so badly. God, I love him and feel I need him. Will we ever be a happy, healthy family again?

Sara is such a good friend with others her age. When she visited us here in Iowa City, she adored Roths' seven-month-old grandson, Shawn. She carried him as if he were her Cabbage Patch doll. How much of their lives I am missing! Oh, I want to be their mom, yet there is no way to make up for these lost days. They are lived. They are gone.

The predictable crises and complications of bone marrow transplant began hitting me: fevers, chills, fluid retention. On day zero plus six, I began losing my hair in large clumps. I lost my mustache but retained my eyebrows. My sense of taste left. Everything I ate tasted like cardboard.

One of my more uncomfortable complications was chronic diarrhea, apparently associated with radiation. My doctors told me I had set a floor record for output—three and a half liters in twenty-four hours! Treatment meant nothing by mouth for several weeks, nutrition through a chest catheter, then a slow rebuilding process.

More serious complications were the bouts with infection. At several points I was on three different IV antibiotics simultaneously. Several of my major body systems, including kidney, liver, heart, and lungs, also showed the trauma of the transplant.

Death seemed to camp out on the foot of my bed. One afternoon I was receiving an IV treatment of gamma globulin, which is a high protein substance difficult to diffuse through the body. Given too rapidly, it can lead to congestive heart failure.

After about twenty minutes of treatment, I noticed chest heaviness. It soon felt like an elephant standing directly on my chest. I called my nurse, who immediately began administering diuretic therapy. Within an hour I had passed the excess fluid, and life was again stable.

For sixty minutes I felt the panic common to respiratory patients. Was this the end? Staff assured me I was not in a life-and-death crisis. I could not receive their words of comfort.

On January 25 (day plus ten) I wrote in my journal,

> Lord, I fear death. It is never very far away nor very deep in the background. Help me to face it, to own it, then to give it to you, the one who consistently promises, "It is I; do not be afraid."

I was in isolation until my blood counts rose to safe levels. I worried only about my battle. I was insulated from the battles being fought and lost beyond my door. Joyce was not.

01/26/87 DEATH! IT'S *a reality here! I feel so emotional! Eddie died last night, a six-year-old who had been here since June. That poor mom!*

Jake made it through the night. I talked to his wife, Amy, today. He wasn't expected to survive but did. He's not out of the woods. Life is very precious, yet very fragile.

In talking to Amy, I discovered that she has only known two success stories with bone marrow transplant since September. Some have gone home but either came back here and died or died in their home towns. I need to talk to Roger.

Yes, we've known death is a possibility. Somehow these days of isolation, this waiting, the unknown, have all come crashing in on us. It's as if a hammer is slowly descending to crush Phil. Will he be one of the lucky few? Will he escape the hammer and live? If he lives, what will life be like?

How can I plan? I can't. I can truly live only today and celebrate the preciousness of life, even this abnormal life.

01/26/87 GOD, BE *merciful to us all. Show us your love.*

We know these are bonus days; we want more of them. Sometimes I get really scared when I visualize myself: a Kansas widow with two kids in school and no significant income.

At other times I see a Phil who can read and write and manage the kids after school but is unable to maintain a job. Yes, I would be grateful, even for that.

I have yet another image. This one God gave me on October 5: a normal, healed, productive Phil.

God, which will it be? I'm glad you, through your people, will be present with me whatever happens.

I was at high risk for infection during the two weeks following my transplant. I was in isolation but seldom felt isolated. We often received ten or more cards or letters each mail call. By the end of my hospital stay, we had over 300 cards taped to my walls. One gift resisted Scotch Tape. A Sunday school class from Wellman Mennonite Church knew that the secret to recovery was an Iowa Hawkeye sweatshirt. I continue to wear that shirt with pride!

The cards, phone calls, and the prayers of church members kept the demons of loneliness and despair at bay. We had many faithful and persistent cheerleaders. I sought some means of responding to this undergirding and wrote an "epistle" to Hesston Mennonite Church:

January 27, 1987

Dear Sisters and Brothers:

"Celebrate with me the goodness of the Lord. In the words of the psalmist (Psalm 103, paraphrased):
It is he who forgives all your guilt,
Who heals every one of your ills,
Who redeems your life from the grave,
Who crowns you with love and compassion,
Who fills your life with good things,
Renewing your youth like the eagle's."

It is day zero plus twelve of my bone marrow transplant. I am convinced that through your prayers God's healing power is being released in my body.

I have been in isolation since January 15, yet my room has remained like an open pasture. Your cards, calls, and letters have been our window to the outside world. We are refreshed and renewed by words of encouragement.

In recent days God has allowed the hospital to become a place of ministry for me. As friendships develop with nursing and medical staff, I have had opportunity to listen to their struggles, to witness to my faith, to be a light among the nations.

Many of you have prayed for a miracle. Dear friends, open your eyes to the miracle that is unfolding before you.

Last night God gave me this promise from Philippians 1:20, 22, 25. I cried myself to sleep rejoicing in God's goodness.

"I eagerly expect and hope that I will in no way be ashamed, but will have sufficient courage so that now as always Christ will be exalted in my body, whether by life or by death. . . . If I am to go on living in the body, this will mean fruitful labor for me. . . . Convinced of this, I know that I will remain, and I will continue with all of you for your progress and joy in the faith."

Isolation allowed time for rest and for reflection. Eight other patients went through bone marrow transplant the same time I did. Some died while I was in the hospital. All would be dead in six months. Was there any purpose to my suffering and the suffering of those around me? Where was God in all of this?

I remembered how Rabbi Harold Kushner answered these questions. Kushner authored the 1980s bestseller *When Bad Things Happen to Good People.* He had lost a fourteen-year-old son to a rapid aging disease. Using Job as a case study, Kushner concluded that Job is prepared to give up his belief . . . that God is all powerful. . . . Forced to choose between a good God who is not totally powerful or a powerful God who is not totally good, the author of the book of Job chooses to believe in God's goodness.

Kushner then answered the question raised by his book title.

If we can bring ourselves to acknowledge that there are some things God does not control, many good things are possible (pp. 42-45).

Kushner's book struck home with many people, yet I could not accept his solution of a limited God. Neither could I endorse the idea of God as a cosmic jokester, capricious and unpredictable. God does not inflict pain on his people.

I resolved that God does not *send* suffering to us. God does not *spare* us from suffering. God does *share* our suffering. God weeps whenever God's shalom, God's peace, is replaced by pain and separation.

January 29, day zero plus fourteen, brought good news: a white blood count (WBC) of 1,700. My counts were high enough to release me from isolation. I could go anywhere on the floor, as long as I wore a protective mask. Joyce was eager for us to take a walk. I was terrified. I felt like a bull who had been penned up all winter and finally let out to pasture.

To celebrate the return of my white count, we had arranged with the hospital dietitian for a candlelight supper. Our menu included roast beef, mashed potatoes, green beans, salad, rolls, and cherry pie. My sense of taste had not yet returned so I ate by memory.

01/29/87 THE DOCTORS *made rounds and disconnected Phil from the machine. He got nauseated but was helped by Compazine. We enjoyed a candlelight supper, with two blue candles and one white candle, marking the return of his white blood count.*

Later we watched a video, Police Academy. *During that time Phil got the chills. We're on a roller coaster. Moment by moment things change.*

Phil cries frequently—tears of joy, frustration, depression, fear. I must figure out which kinds of tears they are and then decide how to respond. It's so strange.

Phil also has so many physical changes. One moment he's fine, the next congestive heart failure, elevated blood pressure, chills. Whew!

How does one adapt to so very many changes or even report how things are going? All body systems are taxed to their utmost when one fails a bit.

Walking had restored my stamina in December. It would again serve us in February. A hall from my unit to a connecting unit was 158 paces. A lap was just over a tenth of a mile. Our daily goals rose steadily. Before discharge we were walking six miles a day.

Things grew steadily better and I grew progressively stronger. Still the fears and threats of relapse and infection plagued me. My February 8, day zero plus twenty-four, journal commented:

It's been such a long road. I'm so ready for some reso-
lution to the crisis. I'm doing so well. Can it stay that way?

Lord, can't you complete the miracle? Can't you give
me the assurance that you have healed me, that it's okay,
that it's over?

*02/07/87 YESTERDAY I got up and went to the hospital.
Phil had a more difficult night with chills. His lack of sleep
really shows. He was very tearful several times. He is psychologically fragile, unsure if he should plan to live a long
time or expect that life will be quickly snatched from him by
infection.*

*He now has life to lose again. What kind of person will he
be? What contributions will he make? Will he fail? Many
questions surface, some real fears and others imagined. I
sometimes feel inadequate in my responses, especially today
when I too feel like crying.*

*Why do I feel like crying? I'm not sure—tears of relief that
this nightmare may end, tears of joy that Phil's health is being restored, tears of sadness and of loss over these days without Sara and Steven.*

Coming Home

My journey home began on February 10, day zero plus twenty-six. Roger discharged me as an outpatient to Royce and Eileen's home. I was anxious about leaving the hospital. My room afforded safety and security. Pills, injections, and IVs were only a call light away. Others made decisions for me. My responsibility was to get well. I had begun to enjoy being sick. Now I had to reengage with life.

Friends from Hesston had given Joyce a round-trip airplane ticket so she could spend her birthday, February 15, and Valentine's Day with Sara and Steven. The trip reminded us both that the physical battles we had fought and would fight were only part of the war.

02/13/87 THIS MORNING I met with the elementary school counselor. He felt both children would move beyond this crisis with positive outcomes and feelings.

Sara is containing much anger which somehow needs to get out. We need to watch for depression. She feels rather alone: Mom and Dad get attention because Phil is sick. Steven gets attention because of his asthma. She's not special because she's normal. I fear she will have long-term hurts from this experience.

02/14/87 TONIGHT I *fixed tacos for supper. All of us really enjoyed them, especially Steven. I know Steven has slimmed down from lowered steroids. I think he's even gotten a bit taller. Sara is so beautiful and well-proportioned. They both have much to tell me.*

We watched a Valentine special on television and then Star Wars *until 10:00 p.m. We pulled out the Hide-A-Bed. After the video was over, it was bedtime. They were both eager to get and give hugs and kisses. Sara has become much more expressive, physically and verbally, of her feelings. I really like seeing this.*

When we sat down to eat supper, we grabbed hands to pray as we usually did. They said, "There's just one thing that's not right. Daddy's not here. So let's fold our hands instead of holding hands."

02/15/87 LORD, THIS *weekend I experienced what it would be like to be a single parent, living alone in this house with Sara and Steven. That's something that I hope will never happen. If it does, life will go on with your help and the love of your people. I believe you will give to us the resources which we would need to live. Thanks, God, for helping me live through some of this anxiety.*

I ask that the four of us can again live together and be an example of Christlike love. Thank you for the physical and emotional healing we are experiencing because of your power and your love shown to us by your people!

While Joyce was in Kansas, things were happening in Iowa. Roger announced I was ready to return to Hesston. My local oncologist would monitor blood levels on a weekly basis. Whenever I left the house I would wear my little blue mask to filter airborne germs. I could meet with small groups, but I needed to avoid crowds for six months. This meant no church gatherings until late summer.

Since I could not thank the Hesston congregation in person, I drafted another epistle sharing our good news:

February 18,1987

Dear Sisters and Brothers:

The doctors are telling us to think about returning home. Home. This has such a good sound to it. Home to be with the children. Home to be with the people who have so faithfully prayed for and stood by us.

God is teaching us much through this experience. I pray that God will keep our minds and eyes open to see and to remember the ways God has touched and transformed us. One learning is already clear to me. God still makes a difference. The prayers of God's people still make a difference.

In nine weeks it will be Easter Sunday.

Easter—the resurrection of our Lord Jesus Christ.

Easter—the promise of our own resurrections.

Easter—the triumphant news that God cannot be defeated, even by the shadows of death.

In my life, in the life of our congregation, in the life of the Hesston community, God has let Easter light shine. Hallelujah!

It was difficult to say good-bye to the doctors and nurses on the transplant unit. We had known staff for only six weeks, but our shared crisis had enabled us to bond quickly.

It was particularly difficult to say good-bye to Roger, who always took time to answer our questions, even when his answers slipped by us. We shared with Roger the responsibility to make good medical and personal choices about my care.

He repeatedly asked us, "What do you think? How do you feel about this direction in treatment?"

Roger created a climate of openness which let us trust him. While he could make no guarantees, we believed his counsel was the best that could be offered.

We began packing for home. We had everything we had started with and, in addition, hundreds of cards and posters. Royce prepared a magnificent farewell dinner featuring Iowa pork and we headed West.

02/20/87 IN OUR discharge interview, Roger and Rob told me to watch Phil carefully for depression. I shared with them my three major concerns—getting back into the Hesston community, Phil's depression, and, as a family of four, feeling safe from major loss.

Our trip home was uneventful—until we passed Eastlawn Cemetery just outside Hesston. We knew that Eastlawn might have been my final resting place. Coincidentally—perhaps providentially—the "Hallelujah Chorus" began playing on our Kansas Mennonite Men's Chorus tape. What a welcome home!

02/22/87 HOMECOMING DAY! About fifteen or twenty miles away from home we both became quiet and reflective. When we passed Eastlawn Cemetery, tears were flowing down our faces—tears of utter joy.

We know we must get to six months post-transplant before we can feel safe and can plan a future. Today, as we drive into Hesston, as we will once more be parents to Sara and Steven, we are full of hope.

As we pulled into our driveway, we noticed large yellow ribbons on surrounding trees. We had not been forgotten. Once more, church and community people showed support with a special welcome home.

Steven was full of hugs and kisses. Sara was more reserved. Some of this reserve was the awkwardness of reunion after two months. Some of it was uncertainty as to how to approach Daddy. Steven simply knew that Daddy was home and that things were okay. Sara knew the story was still incomplete.

02/21/87 AS WE left Iowa City yesterday, Jan Holland, our social worker, tearfully told me, "You didn't know if you'd be going home together. You took a difficult situation and made it a positive one."

God, I am so very grateful for Phil's life and for all the people who made his life possible, especially Roger Gingrich. Before we left Iowa City I told Roger, "Thanks for giving me back my husband."

Thanks, God, for medical science and the way you can work through it. It takes many factors working together for a success story such as ours. It is a miracle! I really hope all continues to go well.

Starting Over

It was good to be home, yet life was not without adjustments. We needed to move back in, both physically and emotionally. The house had a different feel to it—placement of furniture, the way dishes were arranged. For two months, the children had conformed to Carl and Mary's expectations. Now they had to readjust to our style of parenting.

02/23/87 SARA DOES *not seem to have progressed much on piano in the weeks we were gone. I asked her about it and she quickly stated, "I don't do anything well. I'm not special in this family. I don't have a special thing that I'm good at."*

Sara was crying away. She doesn't want Steven to take piano because she is afraid he will soon be better than she. How can I assure Sara she is special?

03/01/87 THE BEGINNING *of a new month. Five months ago tonight I discovered Phil's "baby." Life has changed.*

I am scared when I think back over these painful and emotional months. Each day seems so significant. I know I can make it one day at a time, but more than that I cannot bear.

Sometimes I wonder if I'll have enough energy to finish the day. I am very tired. I get angry with myself if I get to class late, if I yell at the children, if I forget to tell Sara and Steven that they did something well, or if I forget to thank a friend for their precious remembrances. I feel as if I'm living on the brink of a mountain: if one small thing goes wrong, I may fall to great depths emotionally.

I welcomed visits from individuals or groups, yet many people preferred the telephone. No one wanted to be the source of a cold or an infection.

Frequent warnings about infections and hospitalizations were confirmed March 5, ten days after our return home. My Raaf catheter, used for blood tests and transfusions, was still in my chest. Made of plastic, the catheter was an entry point for germs. I developed a staph infection, which required removal of the catheter and IV antibiotics at St. Francis Regional Medical Center in Wichita.

It was a predictable crisis, yet one to which I responded with alarm. My platelet count dropped dramatically. My fever ranged from 101 to 102 degrees. To have come so far and to regress so quickly—could I avoid a fatal infection? What if the leukemia came back? Would life ever return to normal?

03/09/87 WE GOT home from the hospital around 11:00 a.m. Today's counts are as abnormal as yesterday's. I see no significant change except I will do his IV medications at home rather than in the hospital.

I went swimming over the noon hour. During that time

my mind wandered to the "what ifs." What if Phil doesn't get better? What if he dies? I felt very sad and nearly devastated. I'm not ready to give him up, especially when he was so very well two weeks ago.

The world perceives Phil as being healthier than he is and views me as pessimistic. Life can be snatched from Phil no matter what people want to believe or what he attempts to do.

As I swam I cried. I felt anguish. Then calm stole over me. We have today. Whether we have seven days, seven weeks, or even seventy years together, living with this much anxiety will only push us apart and take away the beauty of today.

I need to throw that anxiety away. For now I want to live life close to Phil, sharing these precious moments together.

The acute crisis ended but the chronic problems continued. I had worked hard at preparing myself to die. It would take equally hard work to prepare myself to live again. I was not always successful.

03/15/87 WHY DO *I feel so lonely? I think it's the uniqueness of our situation. Everyone wants Phil well and us to function as usual. Life isn't that way.*

Phil is very tired, with little energy reserve. He tires easily and needs to rest. Meanwhile, when rested, he looks healthy and walks two to three miles a day.

Each day Phil can live is a miracle. I don't care if it takes six months or one year for him to get his energy back.

03/16/87 A DAY *filled with varying emotion! It was a dreary day on the outside and on the inside with Phil. I did get him to laugh a few times.*

How can I reenergize Phil? I don't like to see him so downhearted.

An analogy came to mind: two sturdy pillars supporting a huge heart. The pillars were Phil and me, representing our equal relationship. We were well-educated, physically and emotionally healthy. The heart symbolized our love for each other, our marriage, family, friends, careers, and our world. Together we could do life well. We could support the things we both believed in so deeply. We were all we could be.

Then illness cracked one of those pillars. The other pillar had to support more of the load. Sometimes the heart was so heavy the strong pillar felt it could not bear it anymore.

Then the crumbling pillar also began leaning on the strong pillar. The strong pillar knew it had to get stronger—but how? People noticed the problem and added support rods. Still the strong pillar was ultimately forced to hold up the heart alone.

Now we are trying to become two healthy pillars again. We are slowly rebuilding, hoping to regain strength, yet seeing setbacks. How does one manage through these times?

04/04/87 I FEEL *frustrated when I try to explain how difficult it is to plan for the future. If I knew the ending of this story, I would know how to plan. If Phil is going to die, I'd spend as much time with him as I can. If he's going to live, I want to start branching out.*

Friends say I need to start planning for the future. For a crucial period my life did revolve around Phil. Now, however, it's time to move on and see what I want to do for me.

Living one day at a time is all any of us can do. I realize that other families could also be wiped out. Yet in our situation, sickness, disability, and death are probabilities. I guess it's hard for others to understand.

04/16/87 DURING OUR *walk today, we talked about how to get Phil into the office again.*

At one point he got disgusted and said, "But you don't understand. I'm disabled."

He went on to say that all the things he wanted to do he couldn't do.

Finally, I interrupted, "I don't want to talk about what you can't do. What can you do?"

It is time to take the sick role away from him.

During my hospitalization at Iowa City, I had promised the members of Hesston Mennonite Church that I would preach on Easter Sunday, April 19. My health seemed stable, yet how could I return to the pulpit after a five-month absence?

We found the answer in the children's time, a regular feature of the worship hour at church. As the children came forward, I sneaked onto the platform, covered by a blanket.

Sue Gering, the storyteller, told the children about moths, cocoons, and butterflies. Noticing the large cocoon behind her, Sue helped the children call me out. To the sound of congregational applause, I was reborn—nearly losing my wig in the process!

My homecoming sermon was titled "Stop Being Afraid," based on Matthew 28. With newfound conviction I testified,

> Death is strong—but God is stronger! The final victory belongs not to death but to God. We die not into cold, empty shadows, but into the loving arms of our heavenly Father. Christ is risen; we no longer need fear death. We can stop being afraid.

At the close of the service, Joyce joined me at the pulpit. We had a surprise. Joyce said,

"Today we celebrate Easter—the beginning of new life. We want to share a symbol of Phil's new life.

"Last October, after we found out about Phil's illness, we planned Phil's funeral. I wanted something to symbolize our faith that life *would* go on.

"With our support group's brainstorming, we thought of a flower. I knew the gladiolus would be the perfect symbol for us. First, the very name, *glad*, would communicate the joy Phil's life had brought to many.

"Second, I had carried a single long-stemmed yellow glad at our wedding. It marked the beginning of our nearly fifteen years of life together.

"Third, it would be a reminder that life goes on, but not without nurture and care. For gladiolus to keep blooming, they must be dug up each fall and then replanted each spring.

"We bought the gladiolus for a funeral. This morning we share them with you to celebrate Phil's new lease on life. As you leave today, one of our support group families will be at the door to give you a bulb. Let it celebrate the joy of new life and hope and our gratitude to you for the ways you have nurtured us through this deep valley in our lives.

"These months have been difficult. They have also been a time of growth. We have given of ourselves, celebrating our gifts and our lives. We have learned how to care for each other. We, the Hesston Mennonite Church, are growing, budding, and blooming.

"We thank you for the many ways you have surrounded us with your love. You have each had a part in our being here today. Let us continue to celebrate new life and hope—for Phil and for all of us."

Two Steps Forward, One Step Backward

We drifted into summer. My energy increased and so did my work load, including pastoral visits, meetings, even some long-range planning. I was making progress, but hesitantly. Illness was always near.

I continued to be anxious about the "what ifs." What if that low grade fever erupted into a high one? Did a variation in my weekly blood counts signal something? What was causing my chronic fatigue?

My anxiety made *me* my most frequent topic of conversation. I acted as though details which fascinated and frightened me also supremely interested others. That stance did not wear well with Joyce or others.

05/20/87 As I put Sara to bed, I told her, "If Daddy gets really sick we may have to go back to Iowa. That could mess up your birthday party plans" (Sara's birthday is May 24).

Sara became upset, saying, "Daddy's sickness is just really messing up my life."

Phil's health makes planning hard for Sara, our planner.

05/21/87 AFTER THE kids got off to school, Phil and I went walking. Phil is doing much better, but he denies his progress. He needs reassurance that he is doing well and a firm kick in the butt to get going.

How do you tell someone to act normally and downplay illness when you know he is very vulnerable to illness?

05/22/87 DURING OUR walk this morning Phil felt the distance between us. I shared some of my thoughts and frustrations as honestly as I could. Some of it was hard for him to hear, but it is such sharing that keeps us close.

On May 30, zero day plus 136, I underwent a bronchoscopy (tube in lungs) to explore a respiratory problem. Doctors concluded I had cytomegaloviral pneumonia (CMV pneumonia). This is a virulent infection to which bone marrow transplant patients are particularly susceptible.

05/31/87 PHIL IS very down tonight. He thinks he will die. He is getting sicker, and nothing is being done. I told him I needed and loved him.

He said, "I know you love me. I don't want to leave you."

Phil needs to talk out his feelings. Tonight he seemed so sure he would die. I'm too tired. I can't even cry.

Once more an infection that others could brush off threatened my life. We left once more for Iowa City. Before leaving, I told the children I did not know if I would see them again. Sara burst into tears, as did Steven. We held each other and prayed together.

The shadow of death passed over us. We realized ever more clearly that my illness affected the whole family, especially Joyce.

06/08/87 I AM discouraged. *My sense of humor is deplet-
ed. I am sad. I don't feel like doing anything, not even cleaning up the kitchen or other routines. Plans always change.*

*Part of the problem is that I am not special to anyone. Sara
and Steven receive excellent care in my absence. Phil is
inward-focused and seems unaware of my needs or accom-
plishments. I'm too tired to help him focus on other things.*

*The uncertainty of the future remains hard to deal with.
We must again pick up the pieces and head for life as a four-
some. This roller coaster is a bit much for me. I want something stable in my world and a place to fit into.*

*The expectation that I will always be at Phil's side, an-
swering his calls and his needs, is smothering me. He is doing well. How can I get him out of the sick role?*

*God, I guess I'm just not good at living in an unpredictable
world. I need some stability. I need to be an important person
too. I need nurture and care, yet I feel guilty asking for it.*

06/21/87 FATHER'S DAY. *We had all wondered if Daddy
would be here to celebrate with us. I'm grateful we're together
as a foursome and can share with friends. With the joy there
is the shadow: will Phil be here next Father's Day?*

*We live in two worlds of thought—one of long-term to-
getherness, the other of abrupt separation. We must make a
choice. And we choose a long life together on earth.*

*I find myself more relaxed, tired, and not wanting to think
about the past year or our future prospects. I like to assume
many more days of life together. This is a respite we need.*

06/29/87 WILL I *ever again be a productive person? I long
for challenging full-time work. I try to see myself as a person
making an important contribution in a job. The thought
seems farfetched. I want to make plans, yet I realize that the
best made plans may only be messed up again.*

On July 1, 1987, I returned to work as full-time pastor at Hesston Mennonite Church. For a few brief weeks, we enjoyed an oasis of calm.

08/23/87 LIFE IS *good just now. I love it: a healthy family, bright people with life goals. What more could I want in life but for this kind of health to continue?*
Thanks, Lord, for this gift of life and health.

After ten months of chaos, we welcomed stability and routine. Our relief was premature. We had taken Steven to Riley Children's Hospital in Indianapolis for what we thought was a routine checkup. A phone call from Riley challenged our optimism.

08/27/87 STEVEN IS IgG_2 *deficient, a rare and new diagnosis. This explains the illness and severe asthma we have lived with these past seven years. One doctor is very pessimistic, saying that Steven has a marked deficiency, This could mean continued severe disease and also puts Steven at a higher risk for lymphoma, cancer of the lymph system. (We later sought a second opinion from specialists in Atlanta. They believed that, with proper treatment, Steven had a better prognosis.)*
Steven has not changed in the past two days, but I greatly fear losing him. What's ahead for Steven? Will he face chronic illness? Will his life be short? Can he reach his dreams?
Lord, hug me tight. Give me strength for these days. Help me change what I can and show me what can't be changed. Let me experience all life's joys and sorrows.

The
Dark Night
of the Soul

October and the fall of 1987 arrived. We had anticipated a happy birthday for me. Instead, routine blood
work showed an abnormal rise in my creatinine level.

Creatinine is a measure of kidney function. Normal
levels are .8 to 1.4. My creatinine level was 3.1 and
steadily rising. This abnormal reading suggested a kidney problem. We embarked on a new round of investi-
gations, relating to yet another team of doctors. The
new man on the team was Dr. H.

To confirm the diagnosis, I underwent a needle biopsy of my right kidney. This was to be a simple procedure. When I returned to my room I passed out. I had
developed a significant bleed, requiring a three-unit
blood transfusion. It was not a good day.

The pathology reports were hard to interpret. Doctors in Wichita thought my renal (kidney) failure was
caused by a degenerative disease, membrano-prolifer-
ative glomerulonephritis. Iowa doctors, looking at the
same reports, concluded chemotherapy and/or radia-

tion treatment had caused kidney damage.

Who was right? The correct diagnosis was significant. If it was disease, even a transplanted kidney would eventually be infected. If it was trauma, my chances were good for a successful kidney transplant.

There was one point everyone agreed on: I was rapidly entering end stage renal failure. The rate of deterioration would continue to accelerate. Within four to six months, I would need dialysis.

When I was diagnosed with leukemia, we chose to continue business as usual. This time was different. Kidney failure would mean a sharp decrease in my mobility and personal freedom. We could not anticipate how I would respond to dialysis. It was time to take our exotic trip.

During our two years in Puerto Rico, we had frequently watched the big cruise ships enter and leave San Juan harbor. We had promised each other that someday we would take a cruise.

Joyce's parents consented to come to Hesston from Ohio and watch the children. We made Caribbean cruise reservations for January 1988. The cruise was originally planned to celebrate my one-year recovery from leukemia. Now it became more significant. It might be our last chance to do something exotic together.

By New Year's Day 1988, I was tired and apathetic. My body poisons were rising to toxic levels. Dialysis could not be far off.

Dr. H urged us to prepare for dialysis by having an arterial-venous (a/v) fistula constructed near my right wrist. This would be the access point for my dialysis treatments. Doing this surgical procedure now would give the fistula time to heal before I needed dialysis.

His argument made sense, yet we were afraid. So many simple interventions had gone awry. We conceded to the surgery. It was a big mistake.

I underwent surgery on Tuesday, two days before our cruise departure date. Doctors had assured us this was a simple procedure and would not affect our cruise. But within 24 hours of surgery, I had developed a cellulitis—an infection—in the surgical area. By Wednesday night, I was spiking high temperatures and suffering severe chills.

I entered medical intensive care early Thursday morning. Massive doses of IV antibiotics finished off my kidneys. There would be no last set of memories. The cruise was off. I was on dialysis.

01/05/88 I AM angry! I'm waiting alone at St. Francis Regional Medical Center in surgery. Phil is again in the operating room getting his fistula for dialysis. I'm angry because we were given no information about this procedure. For example, I thought surgery would be done with local anesthesia in the operating room in just a few minutes. Phil left at 10:40 a.m.; it's 2:10 p.m. and no word.

My anxiety is high. Will he bleed again? What will go wrong this time? Why does he have to hurt? He's tired and gets down and depressed. He's not afraid of death, but he is afraid of dying. He grieves his good-bye to the kids and to me.

God, I realize I'm holding on for dear life. I pray that somehow he will live and life will return to what it was before this illness struck. It will never be easy to say good-bye to him. I fear that time is near.

We are both so weary of this medical junk. I feel out of energy to mount yet another crisis. The roller coaster is hard for all of us. Somehow we expect Sara and Steven to adapt and go with the flow. They too have been through too much this last year. They have had to learn to trust many people for care. Mom and Dad are not always dependable.

Who would have guessed they would grow up with a sick daddy? What will this do to their lives? How will Phil's illness affect their sense of security?

[Later] Phil finally came out of surgery. On our way home, we stopped by Dr. H's office.

I needed to tell him how upset I was. He went over his reasoning about five times, explaining why Phil needed the shunt now. He said we were among the one percent of people who wanted information.

Tears continued to run down my face as I relived again and again the day's nightmare. We will not go through surgery again without informed consent. We need to know how the procedure will be done, the length of hospitalization, risks of doing or not doing the surgery, treatment alternatives.

The next morning, at 6:45 a.m., Sara, Steven, and Phil came beaming into the bedroom with a surprise—breakfast in bed. I was too tired and discouraged to make even a small fuss over this special gesture.

Phil left for work around 9:15 a.m. and was soon home again. He had fallen on the ice. I remembered that I had not changed his surgical dressing. I took off the dressing and discovered a three-and-a-half-inch red, swollen area extending halfway around his arm.

I redressed his wrist and called Dr. H at 9:30 a.m. The nurse said he would call me right back. Phil came home after 11:00 a.m. Dr. H hadn't called. I called again and office staff assured me Dr. H would call back.

The call finally came at 11:30 a.m. Penicillin would be called into our pharmacy. Dr. H would look at it tomorrow on our way to the airport. We should plan on taking the cruise.

Phil and I went to Newton to get groceries, medications, and to see if we could find me a formal dress for the cruise. It was snowing hard. The first two stores had nothing.

We then went to "The Bride to Be." I felt like a queen. It was the first time I ever had anyone dress me. I found two dresses, both of which were on sale. My spirits lifted as long as I didn't think about surgery the day before the cruise.

Phil began feeling worse and went to bed at 4:30 p.m. By 8:30 p.m. he was having considerable chest throbbing. I checked vitals as the bed shook.

Phil wanted to talk with Dr. H. I gave Dr. H. the vitals and handed Phil the phone. Dr. H assured him this sometimes happened with a shunt. All was well. He'd see us tomorrow.

This was about 9:30 p.m. For a while Phil seemed better. Then the bed began to shake and chills set in. His temperature was soon 102 degrees. I called Gordon and Delores Funk from our support group. I knew we would get care one way or another that night.

I called Dr. H. I believed Phil was septic and needed to be seen tonight. We loaded Phil into the car and arrived at St. Francis Regional Medical Center in Wichita at midnight.

Phil's temperature was 103.8, creatinine 6.1. Dr. H at first talked only to Phil and Gordon.

After examining Phil Dr. H concluded, "Joyce, you are right. Phil is septic."

Once more Phil was admitted to the medical intensive care unit.

I am so angry! We were told, "This is like a laceration that was sutured. No problem. No problem with the cruise."

Dr. H must have felt horrible retracting that promise, but he insists he was right in putting in the A-V shunt when he did. I'm tired of asking others to help me. I'm tired of having life in an upheaval and so uncontrolled.

At least Phil will be stabilized on dialysis. This afternoon Phil told me he fears he won't make it through this crisis. He wonders if he will ever again have energy. I assured him he would some day, if not here then in heaven.

I asked, "What does it mean to you to 'not make it'? "

He answered, "Dying is scary, but it would bring relief." It's been a long battle. He tried to cry but didn't have energy.

01/11/88 *My* feelings *are on a roller coaster! At times I feel safe. Other times I'm sure I will lose Phil soon. I'm so grateful for the life we have shared.*

I am saddened by the thought that Sara and Steven might grow up without Daddy. Phil has been a good dad, able to handle Sara and Steven's needs as well as I.

My parents took Sara and Steven to church yesterday. There was a special prayer for Phil. Steven cried and cried. When my dad told me, my heart was crushed. The children have been so aware of this crisis. They know Daddy might die. I just hope they never get bitter toward God.

Many people do well on dialysis. They lead scheduled but normal lives. My experience on dialysis was disruptive, debilitating, and discouraging.

Dialysis attempts to duplicate the role of a healthy kidney. The kidney purifies the blood of body toxins. Dialysis draws blood from the body, filters it, then returns the blood to the body.

There are two basic forms of dialysis. In peritoneal

dialysis, a tube is permanently inserted into the abdomen. The tube is then connected to a bag of dialysis solution which flows into the abdomen. The empty bag can be folded and kept in the patient's pocket. Later the bag is unfolded and lowered to collect fluid from the abdomen. By osmosis, the body toxins gather in the external bag. This bag is changed periodically and the process continues.

Peritoneal dialysis allows the patient mobility and some independence. Its constant exchange closely imitates the function of a real kidney. One is always ultimately dependent on the dialysis, however. And there is risk of peritonitis (an abdominal infection).

Hemodialysis is a blood-to-blood exchange. The process requires an access point (usually in an arm), filtration equipment, and three weekly dialysis sessions, each lasting three or four hours.

The access point may be a fistula, an artery and vein tied together; or a shunt, a tube surgically implanted into the body. Two large bore needles are inserted in the access point, one to withdraw blood, the other to return the filtered blood.

In kidney failure, patients seldom urinate and often have excessive fluid buildup. Dialysis helps pull off excess fluid. Patients must severely restrict fluid intake, for what goes in must come out. A weight gain of three to four pounds between treatments is acceptable. My weight gain was often eight to ten pounds.

Normal creatinine levels are about 1.0. My creatinine levels, even on dialysis, hovered at 10.0! The body toxins eroded my physical strength. I got up late, went to dialysis, then came home and slept until morning, taking time out only to eat. My poor functioning was taking a heavy toll on the family.

02/11/88 LAST NIGHT at supper, while Daddy was at dialysis, we three talked about the possibility that Daddy could have a kidney transplant. We talked through the questions. Where would they stay? Would Daddy be in Iowa or Wichita? What about birthdays?

It ended with Steven crying. What if Daddy would die? Steven said he didn't want to talk about it any more; he began watching a video tape.

Sara and I sat in the living room on a rocking chair. She was worried that Mommy or Daddy would miss her birthday. We talked about alternatives.

She said that when she sets the table for supper when Daddy is at dialysis, it makes her cry. "What if it was always just the three of us? Would we go on vacation? Mommy, you would have to work. Who would take care of us?"

We talked about heaven and how happy Daddy would be there if he couldn't live in his body here on earth. Someday we would be with Daddy again.

Sara wondered if I would get remarried. I told her, "Right now, I can't imagine that. I love Daddy very, very much."

Sara does not want me to remarry. I said, "You don't know if you'll marry someone in ten or fifteen years. I don't know either. If I met the right person, I might."

Sara described "marshmallows" in her stomach when we talk about Daddy being sick. She wondered if feeling sad when others talk about their daddies is normal. Would I have such feelings if I were ten and my daddy had a bad kidney problem?

"I'm almost ten!" she sobbed. "I should be helping out more and doing more things."

I assured her that she is already helping in many ways and that I am proud of her. I said, "It's only natural for you to be grouchy when so many difficult things are happening. I get grouchy too. Don't feel bad or guilty. It's part of the mixed-up feelings we all have. No one can be perfect all the time. You're facing grown-up problems, even though you're still a child."

God, it's hard to see the children hurt. The insecurities of losing a parent, the awareness that death of a parent is a real possibility—fears over which we have no control.

I so much want life for the four of us. Can we live that way? Will the bright and beautiful days return—ever?

02/19/88 MY HEART is heavy today. I wonder how long we will be a family of four. These fears keep coming back and grip my soul.

I can't imagine Phil not beside me in bed, not there to urge me on when I feel insecure and insignificant. How could I ever manage the care of Sara and Steven alone?

Many before me have managed these tasks. While I find comfort in knowing that others have made it through, it's just not the way that I want life to be.

03/11/88 IT'S JUST plain tough. Phil just left for dialysis. His tummy is big, he's uncomfortable, he's blah, he has no energy.

His life revolves around getting Steven up, taking medications, showering, breakfast, walking 1 1/4 miles, resting, lunch, walking an additional mile, snack, resting, supper, resting, bed. He's so involved in himself. Life is not fun for him, even on these beautiful days of blue skies, daffodils, signs of spring and birds. He doesn't mind being bored. Even reading a book or a magazine is not enjoyable. He says he can neither concentrate nor remember what he has read.

In addition to my physical decline, these body poisons sabotaged my emotional energy. This apathy was by far the worst consequence of dialysis. The children would come close to me and I was indifferent to their presence. Friends would come to visit and I would offer monosyllabic grunts in response.

During this wilderness period, God was quiet. I knew God was present. I simply could not find the energy to take God's outstretched hand. In moments of weariness, I dreamed about miracle cures or spontaneous remission. At other times, I wanted to slip away and be overtaken by death. Death began looking like a welcome friend rather than an intrusive stranger.

03/16/88 THE LAST twenty-four hours I fantasized how Phil might die. The news is as devastating as the first diagnosis of leukemia. Hope for a life of better health is gone.

We concentrate on finishing life together—funerals, finances, planning for a hospice program. My hopes are crushed. His body can no longer support life here on earth. His spirit is still strong, yet is being snatched away.

I envision lying close to Phil on a bed in the family room one night as he dies. Friends stay with me. When morning comes I tell Sara and Steven that Daddy has died. He's with Jesus in heaven and will no longer be living with us. I take them to the family room to see his lifeless body. The funeral soon follows and with it a final good-bye.

Then what Lord? I'll be a single mom with two beautiful children. Yes, I am educated. I have a good work record. Still. . . . Will there be energy to make the decisions I must? Where will we live? Will I find a job I love? Will people continue their support?

Much of my joy in the last eighteen years has grown out of our marital love for each other. Now our love is threatened. Lord, grant me wisdom and strength to live these days.

03/22/88 Steven is so angry. We had an episode before school. He wanted to take his fishing pole to school. I didn't want him to because getting it home would be a problem. We tried to help him control his anger, setting limits and telling him what he could do and what he couldn't do.

03/27/88 Home has not been a happy place lately. We have not laughed much nor has Phil interacted much. He says that I'm the only one he feels in contact with. That's too narrow. We're both drained. How much can I give?

04/02/88 This was a rainy, nothing day. Phil has dreams of being in a jail. He does not want more tests and prodding, nor does he think he will get better.

I told him, "You're an important person."

He answered, "I used to be."

He's angry at God and the whole world. I don't blame him. He's tried hard.

We returned to the University of Iowa Hospitals and Clinics for another round of testing and evaluation. Predictably, we ran into complications and unprecedented problems. Our plan had been to stay in Iowa a few days. The days became weeks. We had not anticipated this lengthy separation from Sara and Steven. Of more immediate concern was Joyce's graduate program.

Amidst the uncertainties and ambushes of these years, Joyce had sustained her graduate program at Wichita State University in health administration. It was now her final semester and time for comprehensive exams. The exams were to be given in Wichita; we were in Iowa City. What to do?

04/10/88 IN SIX DAYS I am to write my comprehensive exams. Am I capable of that level of thinking? Should I give up all my goals to stay with Phil?

I called Roger and asked for his counsel. He said, "This is not the time to throw in the towel. The really bad things have been ruled out. Whatever is wrong with Phil is probably fixable. Phil may still be a candidate for kidney transplant."

We decided I would go home for comprehensive exams and postpone further medical tests for Phil until my return. This feels good!

Within a few weeks, we were back in Hesston. Joyce had passed her comprehensive exams, and my tests were complete but inconclusive. Our medical major problem was keeping my access sites open. My first fistula lasted less than six weeks. A chest catheter was reinserted to maintain temporary treatment.

My second shunt never did work. My third shunt consisted of a Gortex "rubber" tube placed in my upper left arm. All in all, I underwent surgery eight times to unclog the shunts which are necessary for dialysis.

04/20/88 AT 12:40 P.M. Phil went to surgery. Dr. S came out at 3:25. Keeping Phil's access points open is going to be a continuing problem. Something is wrong with his blood vessels. The second shunt Dr. S put in only weeks before is already sclerosed.

I believe we're in at least as bad a situation as we were with leukemia. Sometimes I don't think it would be all bad for

Phil to die. I wonder what he would look like and say when he woke up in heaven with a whole body. He would feel so good. Now he has holes in his feet and arms and the long scar in his side. His suffering and age remind me of Jesus. How long must he suffer? Can this cup be removed from him?

Our lives continued to lurch along from one disappointment to another. The never-ending surprises and medical emergencies were eroding our resiliency. One casualty of fatigue was our relationship with my kidney doctor.

05/19/88 ON WEDNESDAY, May 4, Phil and I met with Dr. H. We wanted to talk with him about our relationship and to look at ways to improve the relationship in the future.

I explained that we saw him as the captain of Phil's ship. Just now we needed two things from this captain. First, a person I could talk with when things weren't going well. Second, someone to communicate with our Iowa City doctors and other physicians. These were essential needs in our medical situation.

I acknowledged that our history as doctor-patient had been bumpy. Dr. H wanted to know each thing we were unhappy about. I had a list, but I preferred to talk about the times we felt cared for. He seemed to listen to these.

We went round and round on Phil's symptoms. Finally Dr. H said, "Maybe it's time you consider a new physician. My feelings aren't going to be hurt." He added, "You'd better look at this as a two-way street. Give the next doctor a chance. The more doctor-hopping you do, the lower the quality of care you'll receive."

Our relationship with Dr. H ended abruptly, with disappointment for all involved. More flexibility on both sides might have made a difference. However, neither we nor Dr. H had the emotional resilience to start over.

The bright spot of this long night was Joyce's completion of her second graduate degree.

05/21/88 TODAY I graduated from Wichita State University with a master's in health science administration! I had a cap, gown, robe—the whole bit. The whole family—even Phil—was there as I marched across the stage to receive my diploma.

Many emotions fill me. I'll greatly miss my classmates. My instructors have been surprisingly supportive and flexible. School has been a place where I could do something right and feel normal.

God, you've brought me this far. I trust you for my next job and to provide the time and place for it. School was the best thing I could have done with these weeks and months. Thanks!

Dying
to Live

Life on dialysis was difficult and ineffective. Once again our only hope was a transplant, this time a kidney transplant. Unlike bone marrow transplant, a kidney transplant need not be from a sibling donor. Doctors look for six match points called *antigens*. The closer the match, the better the chances are for engraftment without rejection.

I was not a good candidate for kidney transplant. There was the dispute about my diagnosis. In addition, my previous siege with illness made me a high risk patient. With 10,000 people waiting for a new kidney, medical review teams have to make tough ethical decisions regarding who receives a donor kidney.

We spent four months trying to convince doctors to give us a chance. Doctors in both Wichita and Iowa City were hesitant. I underwent a diverse range of tests: chest X-rays, upper gastrointestinal series, abdominal CT scans, cystogram, lymphangiogram, three attempted liver biopsies, paracentesis, thoracentesis, echocardiograms, and, of course, repeated blood work.

Getting on a kidney waiting list was only half the battle. From whom would I get a kidney? Physicians describe kidney transplants in terms of *half-life*. For example, a half-life of seven years means that fifty percent of the transplanted kidneys are still functioning seven years after transplantation.

Transplants from a living donor have a half-life of about twenty years. My next door neighbor, Waldo Miller, has had his brother's kidney for over twenty years. A cadaver kidney has a half-life of about seven years.

My sister, Beth, was an obvious consideration. She and I now have identical immune systems and are a perfect match. There are, however, differences between a bone marrow transplant and a kidney transplant. Marrow is self-replacing; kidneys are not. Asking one person to sacrifice an organ for another is a very different ethical ball game.

The issue became moot when doctors ruled Beth out on medical grounds. They refused to consider anything but a perfectly healthy donor with perfectly healthy kidneys.

I became increasingly dependent on Joyce for even the most basic tasks. For over a year, she had juggled her commitment to me and to her career goals. Fatigue was setting in.

05/24/88 LAST NIGHT *Sara graduated from elementary school. Phil and I went to the carry-in supper. Phil did not feel good. He was a zombie, offering nothing to the conversation. I grieve for the Phil I used to know. I notice I compensate by talking more than usual. I hope that soon he gets a kidney and can be the old Phil. People relate less and less with him because he cannot respond to them.*

It's hard to see Phil doing so poorly socially. I long for his health. I long to walk beside a strong and healthy Phil again. I don't like to see him this way.

Sometimes I pray, "Let this cup pass from me if it is your will. Let him die rather than live many years like this." In the same breath I plea, "I know you can heal him. Give him another chance."

06/13/87 TODAY I woke up feeling tired and sad. I think back to three years ago and life in Elkhart. I was functioning at a high level. The entire family was functioning at a high level. Could we attain those levels again? That challenge is equivalent to climbing a large mountain.

On June 14, 1988, Iowa City placed me on the kidney waiting list. We responded with euphoria. We were fighting each other to telephone friends with the good news. Steven could not wait to tell someone. He ran down the street to our neighbors, the Blossers. He pounded on their window because they were too slow answering the door and blurted out the good news.

06/14/88 TODAY IT happened! We are on a priority waiting list for a kidney transplant at Iowa City. Sara was with me when the call came. I could not believe it. They need more information but see no reason Phil should not receive a kidney if one becomes available. We all screamed—Sara, Steven, and me. I could hardly hear.

I was now a transplant candidate; however, I had no donor. My only chance was a cadaver kidney. How does one pray for such a kidney? My resurrection could only happen through the death of someone else. Someone who had dreams and goals. Someone who loved and was loved in return. Someone who wanted to live as much as I did.

Dialysis continued to go poorly. Life at our house was at a survival level. We needed a new source of hope and energy.

06/16/88 I CAN'T believe how these days fly by. We get up about 7:30 a.m., shower, and eat breakfast. Phil and I walk one mile. I do exercises and lift weights.

On dialysis days I pack lunches and we leave at 9:45 a.m. Phil is on dialysis by 11:00 a.m. I go to WSU to swim, shower, do one or two errands, go back to dialysis, talk with Phil, and bring him home. By then it's 3:00 p.m. or later.

I straighten the house, do errands, get supper, have devotions. I read a chapter for the family out of a Laura Ingalls Wilder book, walk Phil, and change his dressing. Phil goes to bed, after which I straighten the house and do desk work.

Between 9:00 and 9:30 p.m., Sara and Steven go to bed. I fold wash while I listen to the news. At 10:30 p.m., I go to bed.

06/23/88 TODAY WE went on to Eberly Farms for a dialysis picnic. Phil was tired. All he wanted to do was sit, not even talk. I found myself deeply discouraged. How long will this life continue? Remembering our old life, I grieve over how different things might have been.

Phil's emotions are totally flat. He spills food all over himself. He doesn't care about anything. He wears the same clothes and shaves only every other day, often missing whiskers. He drinks too many fluids and eats forbidden food. He has no will power. He's just not attractive.

I try to put myself in his shoes. He must be incredibly weary. He has always watched his weight, been well groomed, and enjoyed people. He's just not Phil.

On our way home from the picnic, the song "We Almost Had It All" played. Tears ran down my face. I wanted to run away and cry and cry.

We have the option to stop dialysis. Is it better to live this way or to let him die? I don't know.

We elected to have an anointing service with our support group and several pastoral colleagues. I had performed several such services. I never expected to be receiving one.

The ordinance of anointing, part of *The Mennonite Confession of Faith*, is based on James 5:14-15.

> Is any one of you sick? He should call the elders of the church to pray over him and anoint him with oil in the name of the Lord. And the prayer offered in faith will make the sick person well; the Lord will raise him up. If he has sinned, he will be forgiven.

James does not prescribe a formula through which people can manipulate God. Anointing is not a power play. It is an act of surrender, allowing God to bring wholeness in whatever form God chooses.

On June 29 the support group gathered in our living room. We sang, we reflected, we prayed. Our prayers were not for magic answers or quick-fix cures. We opened ourselves to God's will, whatever direction that might take.

06/30/88 THE LAST *day of June! Another month is gone. We are becoming increasingly eager for Phil to get a kidney. Each time the phone rings, our ears perk up. Could this be the call? We had the anointing service last night. We are ready to go. Still we must wait.*

Tomorrow I am sending off an article based on my research paper to see if I can get it published. This step is a major relief! We're ready for a kidney, for getting life back together, and for finding a job for me.

Thanks for your support, Lord, through your people. Thanks for hugging us so closely. Good night.

At 4:00 a.m., on July 1, thirty-six hours after our anointing service, a phone call woke us. A young man, age eighteen, had died in a car accident near Tyler, Texas. A computer registry confirmed that he and I were a perfect six-point match!

This was the call we had been waiting for. Was it a dream? Joyce ran downstairs and had the caller repeat everything. Yes, there was a match. How soon could we be in Iowa City?

We called our pilot, Stan Roth, who told us to prepare for a 7:30 a.m. takeoff. For the first time in six months I felt some excitement. We called our parents and members of our support group. We woke Sara and Steven gently and told them the news.

In the midst of showers and breakfast we paused— to remember. Somewhere a family was grieving deeply. Their son's death offered me a new lease on life.

Under normal circumstances, a recipient never learns the identity of his or her donor. Our story includes a remarkable twist.

The Fox Television Network was developing a documentary on organ donation and transplant. Its crews were in Tyler, Texas, when Mackenzie "Kenny" Wilson was pronounced brain dead.

Kenny was a football player for the Bullard Panthers. Only one month before the accident, Kenny had graduated from high school.

Kenny and his brother were returning home after an evening visit with Kenny's girlfriend. Kenny apparently fell asleep at the wheel. His truck smashed into a semitruck.

Six days after the accident, Kenny was pronounced brain dead. His mother, Penny, agreed to donate Kenny's organs so some good might come out of the tragedy. His heart and liver went to two men in Texas. One kidney went to a woman in Minnesota. The other kidney was assigned to me.

To complete Kenny's story, a television crew came to Hesston in November 1988 and taped both a worship service and an interview with us. For over a year, we heard nothing further. We assumed the project had been dropped. Then, during the 1989 Christmas season, one of Joyce's cousins in Illinois saw a clip of a program entitled *Dying to Live*. It was Kenny's story.

We now own a copy of *Dying to Live*. While much of the video focuses on the heart and liver recipients, one section includes photographs of Kenny and interviews with his mother, girlfriend, and stepsister.

I look into Kenny's blue eyes and I wonder. Kenny

and his mother had discussed organ donation long before his accident. Did he have some intuition that he
might not live a normal life span? What would I say to
Kenny if given the opportunity? What luck—or divine
providence—led to his death and to my recovery?

We left the Newton Airport on schedule—Joyce,
Ruth Epp, and me. Joyce had learned the hard way
never to sit through surgery alone. Ruth was a kindergarten teacher on summer vacation. She had volunteered to be our designated friend.

We arrived in Iowa City about 9:00 a.m. Royce was
waiting to whisk us to the University Hospitals. Even
though the kidney was an initial match, additional
cross-matches were required. It was not until early
evening that I received a full go-ahead for transplant.

The transplant team began its work about 9:00 p.m.
By 1:00 a.m. Saturday (July 2), I had a new kidney producing abundant quantities of urine.

In the first hours following kidney transplant, it is
critical that the catheter line draining urine from the
bladder remain open. During these hours tiny blood
clots are passed which can block the catheter. The
transplanted ureter is sutured into the bladder. These
sutures are fragile. Excessive pressure on the sutures
can result in tearing.

My catheter clogged—and was changed—five times.
I became obsessed with knowing that the system was
still open. Joyce monitored things the first night, but
grew exhausted.

Ruth assumed a new title, "bladder inspector." Ruth
sat quietly by my bed. Every four or five minutes, I
quizzed her if urine was still running in the tube. She

responded with patience and understanding.

Several days into recovery, we discovered that a nerve had been damaged or pinched in my right leg. This resulted in numbness and some painful falls. It would be a year until I regained full use of my leg.

07/08/88 I'M CONCERNED about Phil's tiredness and flat emotions. He says he still feels happy inside and thinks he will get well, yet he's discouraged that he is not feeling better.

We made a list of the things going well and those going poorly. The list of things going poorly was the longest—inadequate urination, leg numbness, pain, heartburn, and poor appetite. Things going well included a falling creatinine level, and my presence with him in the hospital.

How do I deal with him? My usual reassurances are not working. He gets angry with me, asking, "How can you think things are going well? You're not the one who has the bum leg. You're not the one with pain."

At least he shows emotion!

I've pulled back from doing much of his care while trying to empathize and be supportive. I want to encourage normal behaviors and discourage sick behaviors.

My discharge procedure was well established: outpatient to Royce and Eileen's, then back to Hesston. I now had the resources for physical recovery. But emotionally I was exhausted. How many more battles to fight? How many more burdens to endure? Every time things stabilized, something else went wrong.

I was weary of the fight. My motto became "I can't." Up to this point, gentle nudges from Joyce had been sufficient to pull me out of depression. Now the nudges needed to become shoves.

07/12/88 YESTERDAY WE *managed to get out of the hospital! Yea! Now we have the extremely difficult task of reintegrating Phil into life and living.*

For six months he has pulled back from life into himself and his body functions. He was too sick part of that time to reach out to Sara and Steven and me. He had little energy. He seemed too tired to express any emotions. People would talk to him, and he would not respond. His facial expressions were often blank, or he would close his eyes during conversation.

The first few days after transplant, he responded like the old Phil. This was thrilling to me. He cut into conversations, joked, was willing to set goals for return to work and life.

Now he resists. He doesn't want to walk for fear of falling. Even when I'm with him and suggest we walk farther, he doesn't want to. He lingers when it's time to do things for himself—bathcare, dressing, medications, putting things away. Sometimes I get frightened that he will not get well. I worry that these behaviors indicate severe depression.

Yes, Phil's body is getting healthy. However, if we cannot put life back together our story is a failure. We're only successful if we can again be a productive family.

I know that I cannot do it alone. Phil and I are partners in life, to do life together!

09/26/88 MY CHIEF *concern is work. I want to return to work, but how dependable would I be? Could Phil and the children make it at home without me? Work is where I would be the happiest—but where and how much?*

I fantasize about jobs that could fit into our schedule. Then something happens. I don't have the energy to cope with both work and another family crisis. I hope someday this tug-of-war will be solved.

Each One's Life
Is But a
Breath

Once more we rebuilt. By late October 1988, I was again preaching. Life was tenuous but stable. The Hesston congregation had kept my position open. Members were gracious, but the medical crises were taking their toll. The congregation needed and deserved more stability in this key leadership position.

I had come to dread October. It was my birthday month. It also brought ugly surprises. 1988 was no exception. My ophthalmologist, Dr. Donald Scrafford, confirmed that I had cataracts in both eyes. We knew early on that my high doses of prednisone, a steroid used to prevent kidney rejection, could cause cataracts. By December I was no longer driving and required double-size type for my preaching notes.

Dr. Scrafford was patient with us. Despite my medical history and the high risk of infection, he was willing to try cataract surgery once the cataracts were ripe.

Two blessings emerged during this time of waiting. Since reading was virtually impossible, I had to draw on my own experiences and insights for sermons. My sermons became more relevant to human needs.

I was also dependent on retired church members to take me on hospital calls and pastoral visits. This offered them a meaningful job and allowed me to develop close bonds I might otherwise have missed.

11/03/88 PHIL HAS been going back to work more and more. He's been worship leader and preached his first sermon October 30. I'm proud of him. He seems vivacious.

He still has a stomach ulcer. His cataracts are growing. His back, damaged by a compression fracture, seems to be improving. His right leg still gives out on him. He can't pull himself up from falls, which devastates him. His abdomen still gets large. His medications often need fine-tuning.

We walk two miles a day, a great check-in time for us. He puts Sara and Steven to bed each night that he is at home. A bonding has once more developed with Sara and Steven. People seem accepting of him. He still has bad days but overall is enjoying life. It's nice, so nice to have a husband back, the old husband who can think and feel and hug and cry and laugh.

11/13/88 I YEARN to meet my own professional goals while caring for my family. Surely there must be something I can contribute to society, despite the uncertainty of our lives.

God, how does my life fit into your plan and purposes? We've come so far together. You've met all our needs. Give me strength and patience. Someday this time will be woven into my story and shall seem a perfect part of the plan.

11/18/88 I HAVE a job! Tonight I talked with Clorice Powers, a classmate from WSU. She has received the okay for me to work on-call in surgery at St. Joseph Hospital in Wichita. December 5 will be my first day. Two weeks in which to get stuff done. It feels right, provided Phil and Steven do well.

Encouraged by my relatively stable condition, we began projecting a date for cataract surgery. Then, in early February 1989, I became extremely short of breath. Chest X-rays, CT scans, and a needle biopsy of the lung showed "something" but nothing clear.

We called our medical quarterback, Roger, on Thursday, February 16, 1989. After hearing my symptoms he said, "Come!" Once again our support group rallied around us. Within forty-five minutes of Roger's summons, we were in the air.

By Friday morning, my lower right lung had collapsed from tumor mass. I was in big trouble. I needed a thoracotomy—open-chest surgery. The results were expected but discouraging. My anti-rejection drug, cyclosporine, suppressed my immune system to avoid rejection of my kidney. Apparently the cyclosporine had so lowered my resistance that cancer cells had sprouted in my lungs. I had lymphoma in both lungs.

There was no precedent for treating someone like me. We were on the frontier of treatment. Roger gave us a research article to read. It suggested a three-part chemotherapy protocol: pills (acyclovir), injections (interferon) and IV medication (gamma globulin).

Roger could make no guarantees. He did not, however, anticipate a lingering illness. Within a month I would respond to treatment or soon die.

We accepted Roger's counsel, began chemotherapy, and returned to Hesston. I was tired but otherwise felt well. I determined to make my "final" days productive. I returned to preaching and pastoral care. I would fight the good fight all the way to the end.

03/08/89 WE'VE BEEN *home eight days now. In many ways it seems much longer. It's been a difficult struggle but finally I'm feeling somewhat caught up. Life just seems so overwhelming and disorganized. I'm so tired.*

Sara came home from school at 3:30 p.m. We told her Daddy had cancer again.

Her face looked so scared as she asked, "Will Daddy die?"

"We don't know. Roger thinks Daddy may get well."

I picked Steven up from his violin lesson after 4:00 p.m. We told him Daddy had cancer. He began to weep.

Later in the evening Steven asked me to write a note to his teacher explaining Daddy's illness. He wanted to share it with his class. He didn't think he could be happy or play with his friends. He would be too busy thinking about Daddy.

When Steven came home Thursday, he was happy to have shared Phil's condition with his class. He said, "I felt like a huge load was lifted. Now that people know, I can be happy."

The lymphoma crisis reminded everyone that my health would always be precarious. It was time to deal with the vocational consequences of chronic illness.

The Hesston Mennonite Church had been generous these three years. They made sure finances were not a burden. They remembered us in daily prayer. With our biological families far away, they became our surrogate family.

There was no question about their support. But there was question about my dependability. During my leukemia therapy, I had qualified for Social Security disability status. My continuing medical problems maintained that status.

My work for the church was on a volunteer basis. How long could a 600-member congregation drift with unpredictable leadership? The congregation had learned and grown through my problems. But the congregation had lost momentum.

03/12/89 PHIL CAME home late looking discouraged. "We need to talk," he said. We sat down on the living room couch.

His last appointment of the day had been with Howard Brenneman, chairman of the congregation. Howard was concerned about Phil's health, about us, and about the church. Three weeks earlier, Howard had no reservations about proceeding with Phil's review process followed by a vote for an additional three-year pastoral term. But Phil's new cancer was making people question Phil's continued leadership.

Phil had mixed emotions—relief that we would decide on a clear direction, anger that he had not raised the issue himself. We were tearful and stunned.

The question of Phil's future led to others. Where do we live? Where do I find work? Does Phil continue in a lesser role at Hesston Mennonite or do we leave? If we leave the church, what would keep us in Hesston?

I fixed something for supper but couldn't eat. We told Sara and Steven that Daddy might not be pastor much longer. This might mean a move. Neither Sara nor Steven wanted to move. We told them this was a family secret.

That night Phil and I talked further. Should Phil continue with the review process? No. A decision to resign seems the only answer. We will test this direction on our own for a while, then bring the support group together.

The Board of Elders, under Howard's sensitive leadership, worked through a careful discernment process with me. We agreed a change was in everyone's best interest. I resigned as lead pastor in June and stayed on through October to buffer the transition.

The decision to resign closed a door on ten years of pastoral and educational ministry. It also opened a floodgate of questions about the future.

07/09/89 Sara and I had a talk last night. We were alone in our bedroom and she began to cry. "I don't want Daddy to stop being pastor. If he does, I'll never go to church again. If Daddy's not pastor, I won't be special. I can't do special things or help with communion or play in Daddy's office. There won't be any more Bert-and-Ernie children's stories."

She was probably right. We talked about the bad part of Daddy's illness, never knowing if he'll be with us tomorrow.

Sara said, "But the good part is that our family is really close. That's different from some of my friends' homes."

Sara continued, "I've learned you can never relive life, or go back and do it again. I'm not going to ruin my life with drugs, alcohol, or riding with a drunk driver."

Sara wondered if we would lose our house and possessions once our medical insurance ran out. I told her we were looking at solutions to the problem. Finances are a grown-up worry. I hoped Daddy would be around and healthy so we would not have a problem.

There are no guarantees. What is it like to grow up unsure if a parent will live? What scars will Sara and Steven bear?

When
You Pass Through
the Waters

Last week I celebrated the fourth anniversary of my bone marrow transplant. I have avoided major medical crises for two years. Some of the ragged memories of the past five years are beginning to blur.

Our family continues to live with the shadow of death just over the horizon. We call it "living on the edge." Occasionally we move back a step or two from the brink, but we never leave the cliff.

We are aware of death's proximity. Such awareness can be a threat, tarnishing our happiest moments together. It can also be a friend. It motivates us to treasure each day. I cannot assume I have tomorrow to play with Sara and Steven or to talk quietly with Joyce.

We are learning that *now* is the time to create memories. Now is the time to celebrate friendships and heal broken relationships. Now is the time to say, again and again, "I love you."

One memory we now share is a Caribbean cruise. In January 1990, we spent a week aboard the MS *Star-*

ward, stopping at Barbados, Martinique, St. Maarten, Antigua, and St. Thomas. The food was great, the time together precious. Joyce would go again tomorrow. I prefer dry land.

Joyce is now director of nursing at Schowalter Villa, a retirement community here in Hesston. Our medical experiences, both good and bad, inspire her to provide quality medical care for persons in the twilight of their lives.

It is still early to assess what these years will mean to Sara and to Steven (whose own health, by the way, has improved and stabilized). They do have some initial perspectives.

In what ways have you changed since Daddy got sick?
STEVEN: It's made me understand more about when people are sick, how serious it can get. Also I've learned if you stick with God, you'll usually make it through alive.
SARA: I think we grew closer as a family. We know how precious life is. I'm not going to mess it up with drugs or something.

What good things happened during these years?
STEVEN: When we came out to visit you [at Iowa City], it was funny. We had to wear a mask. We had a new family picture: everyone was wearing masks. Also one of the happy memories is the picture of seeing you BALD!
SARA: We got to spend five weeks at Grandma's and Grandpa's. Carl and Mary got to be here with Kelly. I got to go over to Rachel and Rosanna and Jen's house [class-mates] because you guys were gone a lot.

Ten years from now, what will you remember about this time?
STEVEN: Probably the bone marrow transplant.

SARA: I'll remember that the people here cared about what happened and were there when we needed somebody. And that Hesston is the best town because they care about what happens to people in their community.

What would you tell other kids whose parents are sick?
STEVEN: Just hold on and keep praying so that God would heal them. If the chances were pretty grim, I'd pray that when I die I'd go to heaven.

Teachers at school could help by explaining to other kids what's happening. It would help if the teachers had some extra activities for them or fun things to do.
SARA: Stick with your friends. If they're good friends, they'll care and won't say anything about the problem.

What advice would you give to parents as they talk to their kids?
STEVEN: Give it to them straight on. Don't wait until the actual sickness. Just give it straight on, have a family meeting, and discuss it. [The open way] is a lot easier on you. Otherwise you're waiting for your parents to tell you and wondering why your parents are acting so strange.
SARA: Tell them the truth, but be optimistic. Otherwise they'll find out and it might get worse. Of course, sometimes you don't want to hear everything. Then parents have to do what they think is right.

Many questions remain. Will I ever return to congregational ministry? What do I do with the rest of my days? My life has followed a path I neither expected nor wanted. Still I am content.

I am privileged to be Mr. Mom. Joyce works long hours; I help by taking the kids to school, music lessons, the library. I cook, wash clothes, clean house.

Cataract surgery largely restored my eyesight. Reading is again a joy. I teach part-time for the Hesston College Pastoral Ministries Program. Occasional speaking opportunities help maintain my preaching skills.

I remain on chemotherapy for the lymphoma. We continue to tinker with medication levels. One ongoing problem is severe osteoporosis. With a calendar age of forty, I have the bone strength of an eighty-year-old man. Even within these limitations, I enjoy today.

And tomorrow? We don't know. No one knows what tomorrow holds. We do know that the one who holds tomorrow will never leave us. We move forward into an uncertain future, certain of God's promise.

> This is what the LORD says—
>   he who formed you,
>   he who created you:
> "Fear not, for I have redeemed you.
> When you pass through the waters,
>   I will be with you.
> When you pass through the rivers,
>   they will not sweep over you.
> I am the LORD, your God.
> You are precious in my sight,
>   and I love you."
>   (adapted from Isaiah 43)

The Authors

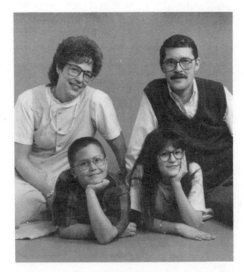

Philip Bedsworth grew up in Philadelphia, Pennsylvania. He is a graduate of Goshen College (Indiana) and Associated Mennonite Biblical Seminaries (Indiana). He has taught or pastored in Puerto Rico, Iowa, Indiana, and Kansas. He volunteers editorial time for *The Mennonite Pastor* newsletter and helps with the Hesston College Pastoral Ministries Program.

Joyce Ann (Eicher) Bedsworth was raised on a dairy farm in Pettisville, Ohio. She received her nursing education at Goshen College and has earned master's degrees from the University of Iowa and Wichita State University (Kansas). In addition to various clinical experiences, she has taught four years in nursing programs. She is director of nursing at Schowalter Villa, a 320 resident retirement community in Hesston, Kansas.

The Bedsworths are members of Hesston Mennonite Church.